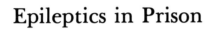

Epileptics in Prison

This volume is published in association with the
Institute for the Study and Treatment of Delinquency

Epileptics in Prison

John Gunn

Special Hospitals Research Unit
Institute of Psychiatry
London

1977

ACADEMIC PRESS

LONDON · NEW YORK · SAN FRANCISCO

A Subsidiary of Harcourt Brace Jovanovich, Publishers

ACADEMIC PRESS INC. (LONDON) LTD.
24/28 Oval Road,
London NW1

United States Edition published by
ACADEMIC PRESS INC.
111 Fifth Avenue
New York, New York 10003

Library of Congress Catalog Card Number: 77-71819
ISBN: 0-12-306550-X

Printed in Great Britain by The Lavenham Press Ltd., Lavenham, Suffolk

Acknowledgments

Research is nearly always a corporate endeavour and it is quite impossible to mention everyone who has given generously and freely of his time. In this study for example there were at least two dozen prison medical officers and many more hospital officers of the prison service who afforded hospitality and assistance at every stage. Especial mention must, however, be made of Dr. Ian Pickering (formerly Director of the Prison Medical Service) who encouraged the project from the very beginning and Dr. D. O. Topp (then Deputy Director of the Prison Medical Service) who assisted with the difficulties of the 2 censuses and undertook interviews at 6 establishments. Mr. Roy Tudor and his staff at the Home Office Statistical Branch undertook the special retrospective analysis of the criminal statistics for November 1966. In these and many other ways busy members of the Home Office staff gave assistance, but of course the findings and conclusions of this study are the author's and should not be construed as representing official Home Office views or policy.

The study was supervised and directed throughout by Professor Trevor Gibbens and without him the project would not have been possible at all. Others who have kindly given of their time and expertise to advise at different stages include Professor Desmond Pond, Professor Sir Denis Hill, the late Professor Sir Aubrey Lewis, Mr. Richard Passingham, Dr. Steven Greer, Mr. Christopher Bagley, Mrs. Joyce Prince and Professor David Marsden. The ratings for violence were conducted in collaboration with Dr. John Bonn and my wife Celia, whilst the epileptic ratings were undertaken with Professor George Fenton. Professor Fenton also advised about the criteria and definitions to be used for the diagnosis of epilepsy. Dr. Pierre Flor-Henry kindly read and interpreted a good many of the EEG's. Both Professor Fenton and Professor Marsden kindly gave access to their clinics for collection of the hospital sample.

Many hours of statistical advice were obtained from Miss Barbara Kinsley of the Biometrics Unit at the Institute of Psychiatry. Miss Kinsley also arranged the computer programming at the University of London Computer. The project was financed by the Medical Research Council, their imaginative and academic approach to this kind of work was obviously crucial. The Department of Psychiatry in the Institute of Psychiatry in London provided more than a research base and a home for the project, it also provided a vital range of academic facilities and contacts.

Parts of this report have been published previously in the medical press. I am grateful therefore to the Editors and publishers of the following journals for permission to reproduce sections of text and tables for which they hold the copyright: *British Journal of Psychiatry, British Medical Journal, Epilepsia, Lancet, Proceedings of the Royal Society of Medicine, Psychological Medicine.*

Many hours of laborious secretarial work and manuscript typing have been cheerfully undertaken by Mrs. Maureen Bartholomew, Miss Kathleen Coomes, Mrs. Sybil Halliwell, Mrs. S. Matthews, Mrs. Evelyn Maxwell and my wife.

Finally and most importantly I would like to thank the prisoners themselves who had nothing to gain, who co-operated so willingly, who only appear as statistics or pseudonyms, but who give meaning to the whole exercise. Most of them have been guilty of serious anti-social behaviour, all of them have paid the statutory price for that behaviour, lots of them have suffered in numerous ways to a degree which is painful to observe. Dry statistics and data cannot adequately describe their plight. For me this study was of critical importance in determining the type of medical practice I wish to pursue for the rest of my professional life.

J.C.G.

Contents

48510

Chapter 5   Illness Factors

Chapter 6   Social Factors

Chapter 7   Discussion

CHAPTER 1

Introduction

This book reports the outcome of 4 years research into the problems of epilepsy that present within the English prison system. Initially an epidemiological survey was conducted to determine the size and characteristics of the epileptic prisoner population. Later a detailed interview and clinical examination of 192 epileptic prisoners and borstal lads was undertaken. This sample was then compared with 192 non-epileptic prisoners. Later still 67 epileptic patients who had no prison records but who were attending a hospital clinic were also interviewed so that further comparisons could be made. The aims of the project were to elucidate any statistical association between epilepsy and imprisonment, to discover whether any such discovered association was valid in clinical terms and by an examination of the differences between epileptic and non-epileptic prisoners to generate hypotheses about the aetiology of such associations.

Epilepsy in its Historical Context

The history of epilepsy is almost as long as the recorded history of man. As Penfield and Jasper point out in their monograph, laws regarding the marriage of epileptic persons and the validity of their court testimony may be found in the Code of Hammurabi (2080 B.C.) and reference is made to epilepsy in the earliest sanitary rules of the Hebrews. Epilepsy has always been treated with reverence, respect or fear (Temkin, 1945) and by the 17th century attacks of epileptic fury were being described (R. Mead, cited in Lennox and Lennox).

Phillipe Pinel, who could hardly have been regarded as reactionary, was able to write in his "Treatise on Insanity" in 1806, that "few objects are found to inspire so much horror and repugnance amongst maniacs" and he advocated the complete segregation of all epileptics.

Considering then the long history of fear associated with the disease, together with the occasional aggressive outburst during an epileptic furor it is perhaps not surprising that when criminology made its first steps towards scientific method in the 19th century, epilepsy was invoked as a cause of crime. Lombroso, the Italian criminologist, who considered criminals to be a form of degenerate humanity, almost a subhuman species (Wolfgang, 1960) went so far as to suggest that although not all epileptics are criminals, most criminals are epileptics (Ferrero, 1911). He suggested that there are three kinds of criminal, the epileptic criminal, the insane criminal, and the born criminal, but that all three types stem from an epileptoid base. He theorised that if fully developed epileptic fits are often lacking in the case of the born criminal, this is because stress, such as anger or alcoholism, is needed to bring the seizure to the surface. His daughter (Ferrero, 1911) went on to explain that "the connection between epilepsy and crime is one of derivation rather than identity. Epilepsy represents the genus of which criminality and moral insanity are the species".

Lombroso has been severely taken to task for these remarkable generalisations. In 1913 Charles Goring discussed the Italian's theory in his classic study on "The English Convict" and stated: "The 'facts' of criminal anthropology, gathered by prejudiced observers employing unscientific methods, are inadmissable as evidence. The criminal type may be the real thing: but if so, it is real despite of, and not because of, the spurious evidence of its supporters; its existence may be scientifically proved by future investigations, yet Lombroso's system will never, by the scientific critic, be otherwise regarded than as the superstition of criminology".

A trifle harsh perhaps, when it is remembered that Lombroso was using the word "epileptic" to indicate some ill-defined degenerate form of man, and was not really speaking of the circumscribed symptom complex we mean today. In fact, as his daughter says, he was trying to suggest that "the criminal is only a diseased person — an epileptic". He felt that "as long as in the eyes of the world, the criminal was a normal individual who voluntarily and consciously violated the laws, there could be no thought of a cure but rather of a punishment sufficiently severe to prevent his recidivation and to inspire others with a salutary fear of offending the law" (Ferrero, 1911). It is clear that

Lombroso was making an early attempt to introduce the medical model into criminology and to take a non-moralistic view of offenders. Nevertheless, the considerable Lombrosian influence meant that the words "crime" and "epilepsy" were frequently juxtaposed throughout the second half of the nineteenth century.

English psychiatrists and neurologists of the same period were also discussing the relationship between epilepsy and crime. No one else took the wide sweeping view of Lombroso, but there was general agreement that epileptic mania or furor could be associated with violence. For example, in 1892 Hack Tuke stated in relation to epileptic attacks, "with the maniacal attacks there is a very great tendency to violence, both homicidal and suicidal". Gowers (1881) had previously described epileptic mania as sudden paroxysmal outbursts of violence to others, usually occurring after a fit. John Hughlings Jackson (Taylor, 1958) described epileptic insanity as usually violent with the violence sometimes taking the form of crime. Henry Maudsley who was, among his many other attributes, a forensic psychiatrist, maintained in his book "Body and Mind" that "whenever a murder has been committed suddenly, without premeditation, without malice, without motive, openly and in a way quite different from the way in which murders are commonly done, we ought to look carefully for evidence of previous epilepsy, and should there have been no epileptic fits, for evidence of an aura epileptica or other symptoms allied to epilepsy". He also stated in the same volume that "whenever we meet with isolated acts of violence, outrages to persons, homicide, suicide, arson, which nothing seems to have instigated, and when upon attentive examination and thorough enquiry we find a loss of memory after the perpetration of the act, with a periodicity in the recurrence of the same act, and a brief duration, we may diagnose larval epilepsy". A later monograph by Maudsley entitled "Responsibility in Mental Disease", discussed masked epilepsy which he thought of as "a transitory mania occurring in lieu of the usual convulsions" and also in this book he discussed how "the result of the long-continued epilepsy is to impair and weaken the mind . . . In some instances this impairment affects principally, at any rate at the commencement, the moral faculties, giving rise to a state of moral imbecility or insanity".

Fashions are fickle; by 1960, only 63 years after the publication of Lombroso's "L'Uomo delinquente" — 5th edition, Lorentz de Haas was able to state at the 4th International Criminological Congress that "serious criminal offences are not found appreciably more often in epileptics than in the average population" (Lorentz de Haas) and that "the problem of epilepsy as a factor in crime should be reduced to its true proportions and not paid any special attention".

This view seems to have been supported by some important Scandinavian work. Älstrom (1950) studied the patients attending a Swedish neurological clinic and concluded that they had much the same prevalence of criminality as the general Swedish population (4·6%) if the epileptic population was standardised for geographical area, social class, and age; although there did seem to be a greater likelihood that the psychologically disturbed epileptic would commit offences. He also stated that "severe aggressions resulting in serious bodily injury do not occur in this sample. Murders or manslaughter are totally absent". In contrast he noted many of the acts of violence to be closely connected with the abuse of alcohol, and also to be of a particularly trivial nature. Of the 30 patients in his series who committed crimes 11 had been violent in this way at least once (aggressive crimes constituted 19% of all the epileptic crimes). Two persons had been committed for several offences. Only in one case was there thought to be any direct connection between the offence and a seizure.

Juul-Jensen published his Danish survey in 1964. He found only 53 patients with a criminal history among 969 at the Arhus Kommune-hospital, a criminal prevalence of 9·5% among the males and 1·9% among the females — very similar to that found in the general Danish population. Like Älstrom he found that the frequency of criminal acts increases with the severity of mental deviation. In addition he noted the crime frequency to increase with increasing severity of epilepsy, but not to be related to any particular type of epilepsy e.g. temporal lobe epilepsy did not reveal any increased frequency of criminality. Most of the crimes were property offences and, again like Älstrom, he found no major acts of violence. In none of his patients was it possible to demonstrate a direct relationship between seizures and criminal acts.

As Juul-Jensen points out, both of these Scandinavian studies were carried out in neurological clinics and therefore do not tell us anything about the criminality of institutionalised epileptics. He might have added that prisons are also institutions and therefore would contain a considerable number of men unavailable to him. Additionally, it should be noted that not all those afflicted with any particular condition attend the appropriate clinic. In fact it is reasonable to expect that those who are disorganised and casual will be the very ones to fall foul of the law and also the ones to exclude themselves from a neurological clinic.

Lennox in his two-volume monograph on the epilepsies (Lennox and Lennox, 1960) agrees with the Scandinavian writers and reports "over a period of 35 years I remember only two instances of murder by epileptics, neither certainly related to the epilepsy".

One of the most comprehensive surveys of epilepsy in recent times is a personal *total* survey of the well-defined population of Iceland carried out by Gudmundsson; he contacted all the hospitals and doctors there, and attempted to interview all the epileptics in the country. He eventually learned of 1169 cases and obtained adequate data on 987. Two hundred and seventy one of these (245 men and 26 women) aged 16 years and over had a police record, 33 patients (31 men — 8·3% or 3 times the rate for the general population, and 2 women) had been convicted of criminal offences, 86 of offences against the liquor laws, and 44 for breaches of customs and price control regulations.

The Epileptic Personality

A complete survey of the opinions expressed between 1900 and 1964 about the epileptic, his personality, and his behaviour would, of course, reveal wide divergences, but throughout there seems to have been an implied association between unacceptable, undesirable behaviour and epilepsy. Clark, who was writing at the time of the First World War, did not follow Lombroso, in fact he went so far as to say "Undoubtedly the (epileptic) character contains little of which one might call antisocial or criminal tendencies" (Clark, 1918), and yet he attributed to the epileptic such characteristics as "sadistic cruelty, hate, penuriousness, pedantry, forms of piety and zealotry" (Clark, 1925). So convinced was he of the existence of a specific epileptic personality that he regarded it due in part to an anlage antedating the disorder (Clark, 1941). Clark's writings had a considerable influence in this sphere between the wars, but by 1928 Notkin was modifying the notion with his observation that "the so-called epileptic make-up is apparent in cases in which there is an early onset of seizures (16·6% of the whole group)". In the thirties Bridge and Diethelm were frankly disagreeing with the Clark hypothesis, although as late as 1944 Sjobring was able to maintain that a specific mental change which he called "ixophrenia" takes place in individuals suffering from epilepsy. "They become torpid and circumstantial, 'sticky' and adhesive, affectively tense, and suffer from explosive outbursts of rage, anxiety etc". Sjobring also postulated that the personality changes are due to impaired cerebral circulation during the epileptic seizures (quoted in Älstrom). In 1948 Cattell enumerated sixteen epileptic personality traits as including egocentricity, vanity, sluggishness in speech and thinking, poverty of ideas, irritability and quick enragement, brutality and ferocity, and proneness to sexual perversions. In a review article Pruyser claimed that "practically all personality studies with psychological tests . . . concur in the conclusion that epileptics do not function as normal individuals".

Hill (1957) and Lennox and Lennox maintained that only 15% of epileptics have personality disorders and Frankenstein concluded that disordered personality patterns in epileptics can frequently be understood in terms of the secondary and tertiary therapeutic and social effects of being an epileptic (i.e. it is not surprising that heavily sedated patients are slow in their reaction times, or that patients who are frequently thwarted in their hunt for employment, and feared by their fellow men are sometimes prone to angry outbursts).

In a comprehensive review of this topic Barbara Tizard discusses five basic theories about the personality of epileptics:

  (i) most epileptics share a characteristic personality,

 (ii) there is no characteristic epileptic personality,

(iii) whilst there is no characteristic epileptic personality a higher proportion of neurotic disturbance is found among epileptics than among non-epileptics,

(iv) there is no characteristic personality but epileptics tend to have a personality resembling that of patients with organic lesions,

 (v) there is no characteristic personality common to all or most epileptics but different types of personality are associated with different types of epilepsy.

She examines the evidence for each of these theories under the headings of clinical evidence, Rorschach studies, animal experiments, and neurosurgery, and concludes that there are considerable difficulties in evaluating the studies and coming to conclusions, because there are important differences between the epileptic populations studied. She maintains there has been inadequate appreciation of the problems of bias and reliability in the judgements made (e.g. clinical and EEG data are often contaminated), control groups are rarely used in the Rorschach studies, and psychological rating methods with assessment of their reliability are usually omitted.

Guerrant et al. (1962) divide the history of the epileptic personality concept into four periods: (1) The period of epileptic deterioration,

(2) The period of the epileptic character, (3) The period of normality and (4) The period of psychomotor peculiarity.

The first period lasted up until the beginning of this century and was characterised by a belief that the majority of epileptics show mental impairment, with occasional behaviour disturbances like criminality. The period of the "Epileptic Character" refers to the time when Clark was writing and featured the belief that epileptics were rarely if ever normal mentally, they were thought to show profound disturbances of mood, attitudes and behaviour such as egocentricity, impulsiveness, apathy etc. These were considered so characteristic of the epileptic that the diagnosis could be justified by such features alone without seizures. By 1930 opinion had changed completely and the "Period of Normality" postulated that most epileptics have normal personalities and intellects although reactions to brain disease, uncontrolled seizures, anti-convulsant drugs, social isolation and rejection could produce defects of personality or intellect. By the 1950's the "Period of Psychomotor Peculiarity" had arrived and authors were suggesting that whilst most epileptics are normal in intellect and personality half or more of psychomotor epileptics have severe psychiatric disturbances of various sorts.

Prevalence of Epilepsy amongst Criminals

Although Charles Goring's important survey in 1913 finally overthrew the all-inclusive epilepsy/criminality theory of Lombroso, Goring was in no doubt that "insanity and epilepsy occur with much greater frequency amongst prisoners". Goring also maintained that crime was positively associated with alcoholism, sexual profligacy, and insanity. He theorised that all these associations were mediated via a primary correlation between defective intelligence and crime.

When Sullivan published his monograph "Crime and Insanity" in 1924 describing the criminally insane population at Broadmoor hospital he found 7% of his male patients and 5% of his female patients to be epileptic. Although these figures were high, they were very similar to those quoted for the mental hospitals of England and Wales. He was convinced that "homicide is *par excellence* the crime of the epileptic" and quoted many cases to illustrate this.

About the same time Norwood East (1927) was urging a cautious approach to the subject of epilepsy and crime suggesting that "the dramatic features of epilepsy are so impressive that perhaps there is a tendency to attach undue importance to the disease as a causative factor of criminal conduct". In spite of this caution he still thought that the epileptic temperament was irritable and impulsive with a liability towards crimes of violence, although he admitted that sometimes employment difficulties could lead to vagrancy and acquisitive offences. By 1954 he had finished his survey of adolescent criminals and had changed his view somewhat because he found the prevalence of epilepsy among London borstal boys to be only 9/1000. Although, as he expected, it was highest among those convicted of offences against the person (23/1000), it was also high among property offenders aged 20 (12·4/1000).

Healy (1929), in the United States, had found the remarkably high figure of 67 undoubted epileptics among 1000 recidivist offenders under 20 years of age (mode 15½ years) seen between 1909 and 1914. It is clear however that a number of epileptic psychotics were included, and sentencing was not discussed, so the material is not really comparable with East's as many such cases would have been excluded from the latter's sample by hospitalisation. Burt in his study of 200 delinquents found 8 cases in which epilepsy was either confirmed or seriously suspected. Brown and Solomon (1942) reported two cases of epilepsy in 20 delinquents under the age of 16 years.

Matheson, studying the reception figures for Holloway Prison (which only takes females), over the five year period 1937-42, stated the prevalence for undoubted epilepsy to be 2·2/1000 and for doubtful epilepsy to be 1·9/1000. He also quotes figures for Brixton prison (males) giving a prevalence for undoubted epilepsy as 8·9/1000 and doubtful epilepsy as 2·7/1000. He noted that about 11% of both the undoubted and the doubtful epileptic females had committed offences against the person and about 8% of the undoubted male epileptics had also done this. He concluded "the irritable and impulsive temperament of the epileptic suggests the subject's liability to commit crimes of violence, the occasional periods of depression tend to lead to attempts at suicide, and the economic stress placed upon the known epileptic owing to the difficulty in obtaining and retaining employment may lead to crimes of the acquisitive type and to vagrancy" (Matheson and Hill, 1943). Unfortunately, however, it is not clear whether his figures refer to a period prevalence, or a reception prevalence, or a mixture of both.

During the Second World War, Hill and Pond (1952) studied 110 murderers electroencephalographically. Eighteen of these patients were definitely epileptic and nine possibly so. Unfortunately the cases seen by these workers were not a representative or random sample of the homicidal population. However, it was thought that they constituted such a significant part of it that the authors concluded that murders showed a prevalence rate for epilepsy well above that of the general population. Morris and Blom-Cooper (1964) analysed all the 764 cases indicated for murder in England and Wales between March 1957 and December 1962, and found eight cases reported as epileptic — a prevalence of 1%. Here it must be remembered that the authors did not examine the cases personally. O'Connell (1960) found five epileptics in a sample of fifty murderers, but his sample was not selected randomly and was probably biased in favour of a high epilepsy prevalence.

In a survey of 532 women shoplifters Gibbens and Prince (1962) only found three epileptics. Cowie, Cowie and Slater (1968) found six epileptic girls amongst 328 (aged 13-17 years) passing through an approved school allocation centre. The most recent survey of direct relevance to this enquiry is by Bluglass (1966). He examined 300 admissions to a Scottish prison and found three epileptics (a prevalence of 1%). The World Health Organisation report on Juvenile Epilepsy published in 1957 reported that Dr P. Scott found seven epileptics among 294 male admissions referred for psychiatric report at a London remand home. This gives a prevalence of 2·3% but of course cannot be regarded as a random sample of either offending, convicted or remanded lads. McCord and McCord (1956) in their study of 325 delinquent boys matched with 325 "normal" or non-delinquent boys found a higher incidence of neurological handicaps including epilepsy among the delinquents (53%) than the controls (36%). West (1963) found one recovered epileptic and one active epileptic among 100 randomly selected recidivists.

These results are summarised in Table 1 which clearly shows the inconsistencies between surveys. Overall the rates vary between 4·1 and 11·6 per 1000, the rates for younger offenders being much higher (12·4 per 1000 — 67 per 1000) whilst the highest rates of all are found amongst violent offenders (23 per 2000 — 160 per 1000).

In brief then, there seems to be a long tradition of association between epilepsy and crime. The evidence concerning this association is conflicting and sparse but some tentative conclusions can be drawn.

(1) The prevalence of criminals attending epilepsy clinics seems to be no greater than the prevalence of criminals in the general population.

(2) A lot of opinionative literature has related epilepsy to undesirable

personality traits, but modern writers are suggesting that this relationship exists only in a few cases.

(3) Although there are very few studies on the medical aspects of criminals there is evidence suggesting a higher prevalence of epilepsy amongst male offenders in institutions than amongst the general population, perhaps three times as much.

(4) The prevalence of epilepsy is higher in young offenders and highest of all in violent offenders.

Table 1   Epilepsy Amongst Criminals
(These figures refer to males except where indicated)

	Sample Size	Overall Rate/1000	Rate/1000 15-20 yrs.	Rate/1000 Violent Off.
Norwood East (1927)	4000	9 (borstal boys)	12·4	23
Healy (1929)	1000		67 (recidivists)	
Burt (1944)	200		40 (delinquents)	
Matheson (1943)	NK 23925	11·6 4·1 (Females)		
Hill and Pond (1952)	110			160 (murderers)
Scott (WHO, 1957)	294		23 (remands)	
O'Connell (1960)	50			100 (murderers)
Gibbens and Prince	532	5·6 (Female shoplifters)		
West (1963)	100	10 (recidivists)		
Morris and Blom-Cooper (1964)	764			10 (murderers)
Bluglass (1966)	300	10 (prisoners)		
Cowie et al. (1968)	328		18·9 (girls)	

Brain Damage and Crime

There is a large literature reporting evidence of links between behavioural disorders and brain damage. Behaviour changes following trauma, accompanying tumours, and in association with atrophy have all been studied and behavioural changes ranging from schizophrenic-like psychoses (see Davison and Bagley, 1969) to anti-social behaviour, have been reported, although it is probably true to say that anti-social traits have been most commonly noted in association with frontal lobe damage. Slater and Roth (1969) in their textbook of psychiatry give a good description of Pick's disease (a form of pre-senile dementia) and reviewing some of the background literature note that the characteristic loss of brain cells occurs mainly in the frontal and temporal areas and that the clinical features include an early undermining of the moral and ethical control of behaviour, many patients indulging in bouts of excessive drinking, sexual adventures, or theft. In a very large series of patients with intracranial tumors Hacaen and de Ajuriaguerra (1956) noted a wide range of "troubles mentaux" which they ascribed to the underlying pathology. In 80 cases of frontal lobe tumour 37·5% suffered with "les troubles de l'humeur et du caractère" a combined assessment of irritability, personality modifications and emotional lability, hysterical states, and psychoses. Of their 75 cases of temporal lobes tumours 24% developed emotional and character disorders. Rylander (1939) reviewed the previous work concerning "personality changes" and frontal lobe damage and went on to study 32 cases in which partial excision of the frontal lobe has been performed because of a tumour or an abscess and he noted a number of apparently specific mental sequelae in the emotional, volitional and intellectual functions.

In Britain, the Oxford collection of Second World War brain injury cases has proved a fruitful source for study of the later effects of gross brain damage. Jarvie (1954) described six cases of penetrating brain wound in which "disinhibition" occurred after involvement of the frontal lobes, one man was changed from "shy" and "not interested in sex" to "garrulous", "immodest" and "constantly talking about sex", whilst another "model boy" became boastful and took to petty pilfering. A quiet but ambitious man lost control of his sexual behaviour after his accident and sustained convictions for indecent exposure. Jarvie concluded that the frontal lobe damage "disinhibited" those areas of the personality where continuous inhibitions are necessary.

Lishman (1968) in a comprehensive study of the same material has shown that brain damage plays a part in the genesis of a wide range of psychiatric problems. He studied 670 head injured patients, firstly using a global assessment of psychiatric disability (intellectual disorders or affective disorders or behavioural disorders or somatic complaints without demonstrable physical basis or obsessional compulsive disorder or psychotic illness) and he demonstrated that both depth of brain damage and quantity of brain damage each make an independent contribution to psychiatric disability.

The 345 patients who had suffered a penetrating head injury clearly demonstrated an association between temporal lobe wounds and psychiatric disability (as measured on the overall scale which included intellectual disturbance). Of the 577 patients who had some degree of psychiatric disability Lishman rated 144 cases as showing *severe* psychiatric disability. For this group the four main categories of symptoms: — intellectual disorders, affective disorders, behavioural disorders, and somatic complaints without demonstrable physical basis, were examined separately in relation to location of brain damage. Intellectual disorders were found to be especially associated with damage to the parietal and temporal lobes of the brain whilst affective disorders, behavioural disorders and somatic complaints were all more frequent after frontal lobe damage, in fact, sexual abnormalities and criminal behaviour were found almost exclusively after frontal wounds. The list of studies relating behaviour disorder to cerebral damage could be lengthened very extensively but such a review would be out of place here. Suffice it to say that there is ample evidence of severe brain damage causing permanent behavioural changes, sometimes antisocial in nature (see also Lishman, 1973).

It is only when minimal degrees of cerebral damage are invoked as producing behavioural changes that dispute breaks out. For example, Miller (1961) in his Milroy lectures doubts the organicity of occupational difficulties following relatively minor head injuries although he himself is in no doubt that personality changes occur following severe head injury (Miller, 1966). In children Eisenberg described the symptoms associated with brain damage as including hyperkinesis, distractability, lability of mood, and impulsive demanding behaviour which is often antisocial, whilst Pond (1961) has doubted the existence of the "brain-damaged-child syndrome" as an entity. The arguments for and against the existence of specific behavioural disabilities being produced by "minimal cerebral dysfunction" are well reviewed in the monograph edited by Bax and MacKeith (1966), although most authors in the monograph seemed to accept by implication the conclusion of Ingram (1966) that "It may be shown that brain damage is a contributory factor in a large variety of different behaviour abnormalities".

Rutter *et al.* (1970) in their survey of Isle of Wight schoolchildren found that psychiatric disorder was twice as common among the physically handicapped as among the general population. However it was 3-4 times as high in those children who suffered from epileptic and neurological disorders. In other words, it seemed that organic brain disorder put a child at special risk to develop psychiatric disorder. They further noted however that there was no special association between any particular type of psychiatric disorder and organic brain disorder.

Social Factors

There seems no doubt that many epileptics have occupational difficulties. Pond and Bidwell (1960) found in their survey of epileptics attending general practitioners in South-Eastern England that 40% had had serious difficulties with employment at some time. The employment problems predominated in the younger groups and the low social groups. These authors also quote the Ministry of Labour as finding that epileptics benefit less than any other group at government rehabilitation and training centres. Gordon and Russell (1958) surveyed 4000 epileptic patients attending the outpatients department at the National Hospital for Nervous Diseases and reported a mean unemployment rate amongst these patients of 9%. These conclusions were largely confirmed by the survey of epilepsy in general practice carried out by the College of General Practitioners when it was found that about 8% were unemployed because of their epilepsy, 6% were unemployed for other reasons, and 12% were only partially employable.

Unfortunately it is impossible to tell from most studies how much, if any, of the association between employment difficulties and epilepsy is related to unwarranted social prejudice and how much to realistic physical limitations set by the disorder. Pond and Bidwell estimated that of the 64 epileptics in their sample who had difficulties 14 (22%) had problems associated with their IQ 18 (28%) had behavioural problems, 37 (58%) had employment difficulties related to their fits, and 11 (17%) had "other" difficulties (presumably some patients had more than one type of problem). However the authors stated categorically that "in no case were fits alone the cause of unemployability". Juul-Jensen (1964) who found the unemployment rate among his epileptic subjects to be at a similar level to that prevailing in

Denmark at the time (9%) nevertheless believed that "a discriminative attitude towards epilepsy is frequently adopted and throughout the ages epileptics have been facing greater difficulties than patients with other chronic diseases". This hypothesis is extremely difficult to test and most workers are content to note the association between employment difficulties and epilepsy.

It is equally difficult to measure whether realistic social restrictions on an epileptics employment potential have important secondary effects on their self esteem and psychological functioning. Jones reporting on the employment problems of steelworkers in South Wales found, in twelve years, 39 cases of epilepsy in an integrated steelworks employing 10,000 men and 400 women. In 26 cases epilepsy was discovered by a seizure at or near work and 3 of these individuals were dismissed. Only 10 of the 39 had admitted to their condition at a pre-employment examination and 3 of these were not taken on. Only 15 of the 39 were unaffected in obtaining satisfactory employment, for besides those who left the firm 18 had to give up their normal job and accept alternative work. Jones, the firm's senior medical officer, concluded, "by existing standards they would be classified as having no employment difficulties, but their choice of jobs was restricted and most of them had to accept work below their capabilities. Generally this work was menial, uninteresting and poorly paid".

This observation may have some criminological significance. Glover and Rice (1959) showed that in the United States when unemployment rates go up conviction rates for property crimes also go up. Thomas (1925) had also come to a similar conclusion in her studies of the social correlates of the economic business cycle. When Ferguson (1952) studied delinquents in Glasgow he found that a boy with a high delinquency rate also had frequent changes of employer.

Psychological Factors

It is a reasonable assumption that pertinent employment rejection and failure will have deleterious psychological effects. Economic and occupational frustration may, however, not be the only burden to be carried by the epileptic. An annotation in the Lancet in 1953 stated "apartheid for epileptics still has power today" and the writer went on to indicate that in his view the two main criteria for apartheid were being fulfilled as far as the epileptic is concerned, firstly he was often kept in a segregated community and secondly he had difficulty in marrying "untainted" persons; the Scots, the Swedes, and the Germans have all utilised laws forbidding epileptics to marry. Bagley (1971) who writes at length about prejudice against the epileptic, has hypothesised that part of the explanation for the familial association of epilepsy and behaviour disorder is that epileptics have difficulty in finding normal marriage partners and hence marry those with mental and physical abnormality whom no-one else will marry. He goes on to lay at least part of the blame for perpetuating this prejudice in contemporary society at the physician's door and likens some of the modern medical views about epilepsy to those 19th century views concerning masturbation.

In view of the possible social, economic and medical consequences or unjustified attitudes in the public and in the patient it is surprising that very little study has been made of this area (unless this lack of study is itself part of the prejudice). However, two interesting papers are to hand, Carter reviewed the records of 165 epileptic children and although unfortunately he carried out no statistical analyses he clinically delineated eight different child attitudes to their epilepsy:

(1) some reported the episodes in a matter of fact manner as if they had no particular emotional significance;

(2) some indicated great concern, and these were usually the children of anxious parents;

(3) others didn't talk about the fits, just the aurae;

(4) many were concerned about the aetiology of their condition;

(5) some expressed anxiety about the effect their condition has upon others;

(6) many complained that their condition and more particularly the overprotective attitude of others prevented them from living a normal life;

(7) several were resentful that they had been accused of "putting on the spells";

(8) some expressed complete or partial ignorance of the nature of their condition.

More recently Caveness et al. (1965) have reported the findings about epilepsy of fifteen years of "Gallup" polls conducted by the American Institute of Public Opinion. While they have noted a clear trend of improved knowledge about, and tolerance towards, epilepsy in the United States, they still found in 1964 that 23% of the population would object to their children playing with epileptics, 21% regarded the phenomenon as a form of insanity and 18% thought that epileptics should not be employed in jobs like other people.

Both Bagley (1971) and Taylor (1969) have come to a similar hypothesis about the origins of the fears and prejudices associated with epilepsy. Bagley writes: "He (the epileptic) is feared because, without warning and in any situation he may unpredictably lose control of his movements". Taylor points out: "If we were without any medical knowledge and observed the phenomenon of epilepsy, we would observe in an epileptic fit a brief excursion through madness into death", both of which are extremely threatening to the observer. He goes on: "Every fit reinforces the view of witnesses that the epileptic cannot be relied upon to participate fully in society, since he is liable, at any time, to go out of control. Therefore, unless he can be cured, he must be set apart; he must be reformed, or else rejected." An individual who is rejected without remedy (i.e. who cannot by his own or by other people's efforts make himself acceptable) has three main courses of action open to him. Two of them were mentioned by Shakespeare, "to suffer the slings and arrows of outrageous fortune" and retreat, opt out, submit; or to "end them", and here it is worth noting the high suicide rate among epileptics (see Chapter 5). The third alternative is to fight back and attempt to avenge the rejection. Burt (1944) saw it thus:

"like other neurotic persons suffering from an intermittent but disabling disease, the epileptic feels himself painfully different from his normal fellows; to get steady work or to earn steady wages seems all but impossible; hence with his unhappy lack of nervous and emotional balance, he is doubly prone to nurse dangerous and resentful moods, and to become hostile to the community that fails to support him."

Lennox and Markham (1953) have theorised that: —

"The restrictions, justified and unjustified that are placed on the epileptic person's activities seriously affect his prospects and accomplishments . . . Repeated rebuffs lead to timidity or to irritations and anger ending in aggressiveness and antisocial behaviour."

No doubt sociologists such as Cloward and Ohlin would have seen the problem in different terms. They would have seen the epileptic as sharing the same goals viz. financial success, happy marriage, rewarding job etc., as those around him, but cut off from achieving those goals by legitimate means because of society's rejection, and the special restrictions it imposes, and would have expected the individual in this situation to innovate new routes outside the socially acceptable means used by others, in an attempt to reach the same goals.

At the present time we are unable to measure the subtleties of these psychological pressures with any acceptable degree of reliability or validity, but this inability which forces us to concentrate on other aspects must not be allowed to obliterate the importance of these interesting hypotheses. In fact they are rather fundamental to the present survey for if we accept that to some extent prisons serve the function of banishing those that society reviles, those that it rejects and those that it fears, and that epileptics sometimes fall into one or more of these categories then it is to be expected that the epileptic is more liable to imprisonment than other people.

CHAPTER 2

A Prison Census

To examine any hypothesis about the association between epilepsy and crime would require an elaborate survey of all the criminal activity in a given community. A court survey would help in understanding the relationship between convictions and epilepsy but even then convictions are by no means the same thing as crime. There is a vast so-called "dark figure" of undetected crime, indeed most of us commit many crimes each year of our lives (breaking the speed limit, dodging our taxes, smuggling a bottle of wine back from abroad, stealing something from work etc). At a glance at the criminal statistics of any year will indicate that approximately one half of all recorded crime in England and Wales is concerned with motoring. Since most epileptics are not allowed to drive, how absurd it would be to investigate a general relationship between epilepsy and "crime", anyway!

In this survey, conducted by one individual, it was not possible to include a court survey. Instead a national prison survey was carried out. Consequently it is not possible to draw conclusions about any relationships between crime patterns and epilepsy. However, it is possible to comment on the numbers of epileptics who are being imprisoned in England and Wales, the differences between the epileptic prisoners and other prisoners, and the apparent reasons for individuals receiving imprisonment.

Two census surveys were conducted, the first a survey of receptions to all prisons and borstals in England and Wales during the month of November 1966, the second a census of all epileptics resident at the same institutions on the night of 13/14 December 1966.

Prevalence of Epilepsy in the General Population

Before conclusions can be drawn about any discovered prevalence of epilepsy in the prison population it is essential to know the base-line prevalence in the general population and therefore a digression is necessary at this stage before the results can be presented.

It is extremely difficult to ascertain the general prevalence of epilepsy with accuracy as samples have to be large to be meaningful, and they should ideally include patients from the hospitals and institutions as well as outpatient departments and general practices; even then some cases will inevitably be missed because the patients are either very secretive about their misfortune or are not in contact with doctors for other reasons. To add to the complexities workers use individual criteria and definitions of "epilepsy".

In a fairly recent survey, Krohn (1961) cites figures varying from 0·9/1000 of the population to 5·1/1000. He himself studied Northern Norway by personal contact with the doctors serving the population and was able to estimate the total "number of people who have problems of epilepsy that need the attention of physicians or hospitals". By this means he was able to discern 2·3/1000 epileptics (53% males, 46% females), with a maximal prevalence between 10 and 25 years. This is very similar to the 2·4/1000 cases estimated in England some 21 years earlier by Fox (1939) who had surveyed voluntary associations, public assistance committees, hospitals and "private persons" in Ipswich. Himler and Raphael (1945) found a much lower prevalence among Michigan college students; presumably low on account of preselection procedures. Stein (1933) conducted a short review of the literature up to that time and concluded that a prevalence figure of about 3/1000 was the likeliest. A more recent British survey conducted by the Registrar General's Office (Logan and Cushion) reports a one year survey in which the number of persons consulting a general practitioner at least once during the year for epilepsy was found to be 3·3/1000 with again a slight excess of males and a maximal prevalence between the ages of 15 and 45 years. Other surveys are listed in Table 2 which demonstrates the variability of these estimates.

Kurland (1959/60) interviewed all the physicians in Rochester, Minnesota, and ascertained that all patients with convulsive disorders were referred, at some stage, to the Mayo clinic where he was working. He therefore surveyed the clinic's records for a 10-year period and added up all the patients who had had 2 or more convulsive episodes. Two hundred and ninety five such cases were found, 109 of them living

Table 2   Prevalence of Epilepsy in the General Population

Date of Publ.	Sample	Sample size	rate/1000	Ref.
1923	USA Draftees (males)	2,500,000	5·2	cit. Krohn, 1961
1936	Michigan	73,000	2·1	cit. Krohn, 1961
1939	Ipswich	92,000	2·4	Fox, 1939
1940	Students (Michigan)	118,532	0·6	Himler and Raphael, 1945
1940	Bornholm	45,000	0·9	cit. Krohn, 1960
1942	Finland	450,000	1·0	Kaila, 1942
1954	U.S.A. (children)	NK	5	Lesser and Hunt, 1954
1955	USA Draftees (males)	NK	5	WHO Report on Juv. Ep.
1955	Dutch Draftees (males)	NK	5	WHO Report on Juv. Ep.
1958	Eng. & Wales	180,060	3·5	Logan and Cushion, 1958
1959	Rochester, Minn.	30,000	*3·8	Kurland, 1959/60
1960	Eng. & Wales (males)	139,234	*4·5	College of G.P.'s, 1960
1960	S.E. England	38,500	6·2	Pond et al., 1960
1961	N. Norway	416,000	2·3	Krohn, 1963
1966	Iceland	177,892	*3·6	Gudmundsson, 1966
1966	Carlisle, England	71,101	5·5	Brewis et al., 1966

*Further details of these studies are given in the text. The figures refer to total populations (males and females) except where stated.

in the community on his "prevalence day". Adjusting the rates for age to correspond with the total U.S. population he calculated a prevalence of 3·8 epileptics/1000 persons (males and females).

The following year saw the publication of two large-scale and important British surveys. The College of General Practitioners collected data over the course of 12 months from 67 different general practices in England and Wales. Unfortunately they do not specify at what point in time they determined their prevalence rate. They seem to have counted all the patients during the survey year who had repeated fits or who had been under continuous treatment for fits within two years of the start of the survey. This number was expressed as a proportion of the population at risk during the survey year. They estimated 4·2 epileptics per 1000 population (4·5 males and 4·0 females) but clearly they had omitted institutionalised and unregistered patients.

48510

A rather similar survey by Pond, Bidwell and Stein (1960) who sampled 14 general practices in the south east of England found a higher prevalence—6·2/1000 (males and females). They defined an epileptic as a patient who had had epileptic fits of any sort at some time during the two years prior to the survey, or who had been on regular anticonvulsants during this period. Again they seemed to have used the prevalence estimate method chosen by the College of General Practitioners of expressing the total number of epileptics found in one year as a proportion of the estimated population at risk. They comment on their surprisingly high result (the highest ever recorded for a general population survey) but have no readily available explanation for this. It is probably best explained by examining the process of selecting the general practices; these were volunteers of the College of General Practitioners, and the authors showed that 3 of the 14 had a special interest in epilepsy and had managed to collect many more epileptics than other doctors. If these 3 practices are omitted from the calculation the prevalence drops to 5·5/1000. The variability of prevalence from practice to practice was ranged from 3·0/1000 to 12·9/1000.

The British Epilepsy Association usually quotes the round figure of 5/1000 as the overall prevalence of epilepsy in Great Britain and from the figures quoted above this would seem a reasonable estimate. In the current research the College of General Practitioners' figures are used for comparison because they are considered to give the better estimate of the British figures.

Gudmundsson's Icelandic survey (1966) has already been referred to (p. 5). He travelled throughout his country obtaining information about all the epileptics known to doctors, hospitals and the social services, and he eventually obtained satisfactory information for 987 cases. In these cases were included all Icelanders who had had seizures or other paroxysmal transitory disturbances of function of the brain at some time during their lives except those who had had only febrile convulsions, convulsions occurring exclusively in association with indulgence in alcohol, convulsions with acute encephalopathy, convulsions or unconsciousness regarded as simple syncope, convulsions occurring during abstinence, hysterical fits, cardiovascular syndromes, and convulsions due to metabolic disorders. Gudmundsson examined 90% of the patients himself. In spite of the relatively broad definition which meant that 56 cases who had only ever had one seizure, and 57 with only two seizures were included, he obtained a prevalence of 3·6/1000 on January 1 1960, and 3·4/1000 on December 31 1964, figures much closer to those of Kurland, than to those of Pond, Bidwell and Stein.

The latest British survey was part of a general neurological survey carried out at Carlisle in 1966. All hospital records, all general practitioners and all school records were examined; a random sample of households was also interviewed. The worker defined epilepsy as "more than one attack of cerebral origin in which there is a disturbance of movement, feeling, behaviour, or consciousness". Patients who had more than one definite epileptic attack were included even if they were symptom free and untreated, which is a very wide definition of epilepsy indeed; some would say much too wide. Even so they only discovered a prevalence of 5·5/1000, which would clearly be reduced if the one fit cases were excluded.

November Reception Census

The first question to be asked in this project was, how many epileptics are being sent to prisons and borstals, and what proportion of the total receptions do they form. A circular letter was sent out to the 101 prisons, borstals and detention centres operating in October 1966 with a request to the medical officers or their deputies to complete a short pro-forma about each epileptic man or woman received into their care during the month of November. By this means it was hoped to ascertain the total number of epileptic and doubtfully epileptic receptions in both the remanded and the convicted categories for that particular month. Unfortunately the estimates of remanded prisoners were later shown to be unreliable. Recording errors were made as the men progressed through their frequent admissions and re-admissions to various institutions. Fortunately no difficulties of this type were encountered with the sentenced men and visits to one or two prisons during the census month indicated that these returns were likely to be reliable. In addition by a careful process of follow up telephone calls it was eventually possible to obtain a census return from every Home Office institution throughout England and Wales.

During the month 46 sentenced men and 2 sentenced women, diagnosed by the prison doctors as epileptic or doubtfully epileptic were received (Table 3).

Clearly there are too few female epileptics for conclusions to be drawn and so the remainder of this study will deal with males.

Table 3   Epileptic Receptions (Sentenced)

	Males	Females	Total
Undoubted	32	1	33
Doubtful	14	1	15
Total	46	2	48

Broken down into age groups and offence groups it can be seen that the majority of sentenced male epileptics are under 30 years and are thieves (Table 4).

The categories of offence which are used in this tabulation are based on codings supplied by the Home Office and are as follows:

Larceny: Breaking and entering. Aggravated larceny. Simple larceny. Receiving. Stealing. Taking motor vehicles.

Fraud: This also includes false pretences.

Violence: Violence against the person. Assault. Malicious damage. Cruelty to children. Homicide. Possessing an offensive weapon.

Sex: Buggery and attempts. Offences against females. Bigamy. Indecent exposure. Brothel keeping. Soliciting for prostitution. Gross indecency with children.

Drink: Drunkenness offences, without offences in other categories at the same time.
(see Crim. Stats. (1966) for full list)

Table 4   Sentenced Epileptic Receptions (Male)—November 1966

Age Group	Offences						Total	
	Larceny	Fraud	Violence	Sex	Drink	Others		
15-19	11	0	2	0	0	0	13	(28%)
20-29	12	0	2	0	1	0	15	(33%)
30-39	4	0	1	0	0	3	8	(17%)
40-49	1	1	1	0	2	2	7	(15%)
50 +	0	0	1	0	1	0	2	(4%)
NK	0	0	1	0	0	0	1	(2%)
All	28 (61%)	1 (2%)	8 (18%)	0	4 (9%)	5 (11%)	46 (100%)	

Basic Medical Data

Table 5 sets out the basic medical data which were reported on the original survey form. This illustrates that prison medical officers place considerable reliance on a previous history of taking anticonvulsants (anti-epilepsy drugs) and a previous EEG* examination. Seven of the twelve men who had never had an EEG examination comprised over half of the 'doubtful' category. It is interesting that in spite of this, over half of the epileptic prisoners reported never having attended an outside clinic; many of these had had their epilepsy investigations within the penal or educational system.

Table 5   Basic Medical Data for November 1966
Reception Sample (*n* = 46 with 1NK)

	Nos.	%
Attended hospital clinic	20	45
Previous EEG	33	73
Anticonvulsants outside	36	78
,, inside	40	87
,, never	5	11

To enable a calculation of prevalence in various categories of age and type of crime the Home Office Statistical Branch made a special search giving the total number of prisoners, borstal lads, and detainees for the census month. The figures are given in Tables 6 and 7 which can be compared with those already quoted in Table 4. They reported receiving 5,096 males and 225 females at the beginning of their sentences during those 30 days.

We are now in a position to ask the first of several important questions. Is the prevalence of epilepsy in this prison and borstal reception population different from that in the general population? Table 8 expresses the total numbers of epileptic receptions as a proportion of the total receptions at 8·8/1000 males and 8·9/1000 females a higher prevalence than in any of the general population surveys. In particular the prevalence is twice that of the GP survey of 1960 (difference significant at the 0·5% level for males).

---

*EEG is a standard abbreviation for electroencephalogram which is a paper record of the electrical activity of the brain as monitored by electrodes placed on the skull.

Table 6 Total November Receptions (Sentenced) 1966—Males

Age Groups	Larceny	Fraud	Violence	Sex	Drink	Others	Total
14	3	0	1	0	0	1	5
15-19	457	11	63	19	2	83	635 (12%)
20-29	1479	58	282	83	42	440	2384 (47%)
30-39	557	48	134	51	88	172	1050 (21%)
40-49	274	52	41	32	126	103	628 (12%)
50 +	156	29	25	21	101	62	394 (8%)
All	2926 (58%)	198 (4%)	546 (11%)	206 (4%)	359 (7%)	861 (17%)	5096 (100%)

Table 7 Total November Receptions (Sentenced) 1966—Females

Age Groups	Larceny	Fraud	Violence	Sex	Drink	Others	Total
15-19	20	1	2	3	0	3	29 (13%)
20-29	38	3	7	29	0	11	88 (39%)
30-39	23	1	6	5	5	3	43 (19%)
40-49	10	3	4	4	10	2	33 (15%)
50 +	9	0	4	2	16	1	32 (15%)
All	100 (44%)	8 (4%)	23 (10%)	43 (19%)	31 (14%)	20 (9%)	225 (100%)

Table 8   Receptions—November 1966—Prevalence Rates per 1000

	Males	Females
Undoubted	6·3	4·5
Doubtful	2·5	4·5
Total	8·8	8·9

Another way of posing this question is, are epileptics more likely to go to prison than other members of the population? The answer here involves a more complicated process beginning with calculating the risk for someone in the general population to be sent to gaol. Although it is not entirely satisfactory the method available on this occasion was to calculate the expected numbers of epileptics in the population by using the College of General Practitioners' estimates and apply them to the total England and Wales population figures obtained from the general census of 1961 (General Register Office, 1964). This indicates that during the month in question 0·72/1000 of the epileptic male population over 15 were going to prison compared with only 0·35/1000 of the general male population (Table 9).

Table 9   Comparison of Prisoner Prevalence in Epileptics and in the General Population (Males)

Age	Epileptics			General Population		
	Total (estimate)	In Prison	Rate/1000	Total	In Prison	Rate/1000
15-24	17,881	23	1·29	3,051,400	2,014	0·66
25-34	21,616	11	0·51	3,944,500	1,597	0·41
35-44	14,625	6	0·41	3,124,900	817	0·26
45-64	10,160	6	0·59	3,135,900	169	0·05
All	64,282	46	0·72*	13,256,700	4,597	0·35*

*Comparing these 2 proportions $d = 7·46$ $p < 0·1 \times 10·8$ (e.g. Bailey test 10)

Age

Epilepsy and crime are both phenomena which are associated with the earlier years of life, it is quite possible therefore that the excess prevalence of epilepsy is related to an intervening age factor. Table 10

Table 10   This Survey compared with the College of General Practitioners'
Survey (1960)

	Present Study			GP Study 1960			
Age	Eps.	Total Sentenced	Rate/ 1000	Eps.	Pts.	Rate/ 1000	Sig.
15-24	23	2014	11·4	104	17,738	5·9	$p<0·01$
25-34	11	1597	6·9	107	19,521	5·5	NS
35-44	6	817	7·3	94	20,091	4·7	NS
45-64	6	627	9·6	119	34,781	3·4	$p<0·05$
65 +	0	41	—	54	13,311	4·1	
All	46	5096	9·0	478	105,442	4·5	$p<0·0005$

gives the age breakdown available in the College of General Practitioners' report and shows that in spite of the expected high prevalence
of epilepsy in the prisoners aged 15-24 it is precisely that group which
is particularly vulnerable to imprisonment. The 45-64 year group also
shows a similar increased vulnerability. If the rates of epilepsy per 1000
prison population are compared with similar raw data from the
College of General Practitioners' Survey these points are confirmed.
Figure 1 illustrates this better in diagrammatic form.

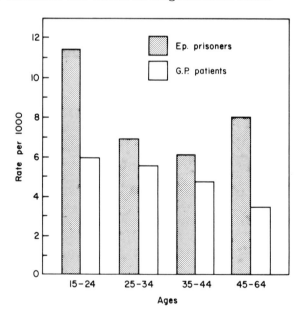

Patterns of Crime

Using the Home Office data mentioned above it was possible to examine the types of offence for which the men were currently convicted during the census month, this is shown in Table 11. None of the differences is significant. The overall pattern is that epileptic offenders like other offenders are usually sent to prison because of property crimes.

Table 11   Current Offences—November 1966

	Epileptics	Total non-epileptics sentenced
Larceny	28 (61%)	2898 (57%)
Fraud	1 (2%)	197 (4%)
Violence	8 (17%)	538 (11%)
Sex	0	206 (4%)
Drink	4 (9%)	355 (7%)
Others	5 (11%)	856 (17%)
Total	46	5050

Single Night Resident Census (December 1966)

A total residents' census was undertaken at midnight December 13th-14th 1966. A simple form was circulated to all the 101 prisons and borstals with the request that the name of each epileptic resident at the time stated should be recorded together with the total number of inmates resident at the same moment. Once more by means of a careful telephone follow-up it was possible to obtain a nearly complete response (99 institutions replied).

The totals and the estimated point prevalence are shown in Table 12 where the striking feature is the close comparison with the prevalence figures for the reception census (Table 8).

This similarity suggests that the epileptics are receiving sentences which are similar in length to those obtained by non-epileptics. If, for example, epileptics had been receiving longer sentences they would have gradually accumulated in prison and been over-represented in a resident sample.

Table 12 Sentenced Epileptic Prisoners (male and female) resident
on one night in December 1966

	Numbers	Rate/1000
Undoubted epileptics	190	6·1
Doubtful epileptics	81	2·6
Total epileptics	271	8·7

Total prisoners = 30,993

To check this point the November census returns were re-examined
in terms of sentence lengths. Unfortunately the special breakdown of
receptions provided by the Home Office for November 1966 did not
include an analysis of sentences. The overall sentencing figures for that
year were, therefore, obtained from the annual published statistics
(Home Office, 1967) and reduced in the proportion

$$\frac{\text{total Nov. figs. (5096)}}{\text{total 1966 figs. (53129)}}$$

to give an expected value for each sentence category.

This is shown in Table 13 which demonstrates that although fewer
epileptics are going to detention centres, a reflection of Home Office
policy, the differences do not reach statistical significance.

Table 13   Sentence Lengths

Sentences	Epileptics Nov. 1966	Estimated Number of Non-Epileptics	Estimated Total Number of Sentenced Men
Detention Centre	3 (6·5%)	734 (14·6%)	742
Borstal	6 (13·0%)	475 (9·4%)	481
0-6 months	22 (47·8%)	2708 (53·6%)	2730
7-12 months	5 (10·9%)	408 (8·1%)	413
Over 1 year	10 (21·7%)	720 (14·3%)	730
Total	46 (100%)	5050 (100%)	5096

$X^2 = 2·9$ (3 d.f.) NS (amalgamating Detention Centre and Borstal)

Conclusions

The prevalence of epilepsy in the general population is about 5 per
1000 whereas a one month census of men received for custodial
punishment in England and Wales revealed 8·8 epileptics per 1000

men. This high prevalence was clearly not due to an artefact produced by the youth of the prison sample. In fact it is the younger epileptics and those over 45 years who are particularly over-represented in prison or borstal.

The epileptics were not significantly more likely to have been convicted of violence offences than other prisoners and therefore violence is unlikely to be the variable linking epilepsy with imprisonment.

Over half of the men coming into the reception census claimed never to have attended a health service clinic for their epilepsy; 27% had probably never had an EEG, and 20% were receiving no anticonvulsants before reception into prison.

A further census of men resident in borstal and prison carried out at one point in time, revealed 8·7 epileptics per 1000 prisoners. This finding suggests that the epileptic prisoners were receiving similar sentences to the non-epileptics. This point was confirmed by further analysis.

Throughout these calculations both definite and doubtful epileptics have been included in the analysis. Therefore before these conclusions can be discussed with confidence the possibility of a bias introduced by a tendency for the prison medical staff to use less rigid diagnostic criteria than those applied during the general population studies must be excluded. One of the aims of the interview and clinical study which follows was to estimate any such bias.

CHAPTER 3

Survey Methods

The next task was to review, by as complete a clinical technique as time and circumstances would allow, a representative sample of the resident epileptic population and compare them with a matched sample of the resident non-epileptic population. In this way it was hoped to clear up the crucial diagnostic issue raised at the end of the previous chapter, and, to enumerate the ways in which the epileptic prisoners differ from their non-epileptic counterparts.

Pilot Studies

The main purposes of the first pilot study were (a) to familiarise the interviewer with the techniques of interviewing men in custody, (b) to learn what problems the prisoners and the prison medical officers felt to be of importance when considering epilepsy and epileptics, (c) to construct a practical questionnaire and (d) to see if any very obvious differences between the epileptics and a random group of controls suggested themselves in the preliminary stages.

Fifteen epileptic boys and fifteen randomly picked controls were interviewed, at Ashford Remand Centre, about their criminal records, present offence, family history, childhood, school history, work history, social history, sexual history, physical health, past head injuries, mental health, fits, and treatment. In addition a short physical examination and a short mental examination were conducted.

The epileptics appeared to be heavier drinkers, exhibit abnormal mental states more frequently and show a greater tendency towards attempted suicide, but analysing the data statistically no significant differences were found between the probands and the controls on any of these criteria, which is not surprising for such small groups.

Following this work a second modification of the item sheet was constructed and three further prisoners were interviewed at Brixton Prison. A third draft was tested on another five men at Wandsworth Prison.

After the fourth and final modification of the item sheet the author and Dr. Topp from the Prison Medical Department began the interview study proper at Wandsworth Prison. A few of the early interviews were conducted together so that we could obtain some consistency in interview technique.

Selection of Cases

The main study was begun in February 1967, and completed in January 1968. It was decided that one or other of the interviewers should visit a wide cross section of the penal establishments in England and Wales and that both the order of visit and the day of visit were to be randomised.

Not every prison or borstal could be visited and therefore a selection was made using the results of the initial residents' census. We chose to visit *all* institutions who reported 4 or more definite or doubtful epileptic residents on December 13th, 1966; this involved trips to 21 establishments. In addition another 9 prisons of the type which take fewer (and perhaps different) epileptics which could be reached conveniently were also visited. Because the visits were randomised there was no bias towards over-representation of any particular region, nor of visiting any region at any one time of the year, nor of collecting the samples on any particular day of the week.

On arrival at each institution a spot census was held, in collaboration with the medical and hospital staff, of *all* the epileptics and doubtful epileptics present at that time, and these men formed the probands for that particular institution. Case selection by this method gave a series of one day samples throughout the country.

After this spot census had been taken an equal number of non-epileptics was also selected to form a control group. These were selected as the next prisoner to each proband in the current numerical index file, the "next" being defined as the card above or the card below the proband card alternately. In this way the controls were initially matched for the probands for sex, institution, and length of time in that particular prison or borstal. This matching for institution could also be expected to produce, coincidentally, matching for age, length of sentence and type of crime (similar types of offenders on similar length sentences are usually housed together) and this is confirmed by the between group comparisons presented later.

The samples obtained could not all be dealt with on the first day and so the interviews were conducted over the next few days, taking care to interview men with an impending discharge first. Once or twice, however, a prisoner was discharged before he could be interviewed, in which case he was dropped from the study as was his control. If the control of an already interviewed proband was missed then another control case was selected by returning to the numerical index file and finding the "next" card still available; this only happend three times.

By this method 192 probands were obtained and a comparison with the one day census indicates that this represents approximately 70% of a one day's expected sample spread throughout one year.

The Interview

There are marked differences between interviewing patients in a hospital or outpatient setting and a prison setting. Prisoners frequently assume that whatever happens in prison is part of their punishment or will affect their future management. In addition, many of them are suspicious of research or of being used as a 'guinea-pig' they feel that any interview conducted with them should be for their direct benefit. Prisons and borstals inevitably contain many individuals with marked personality difficulties, and a number of men had to be reassured that the interviewer was not a "spy" sent from the Home Office or a "disguised policeman" trying to trick the prisoner. Sometimes prisoners are on piece-work and an hour or two away from this means a loss of wages. Finally the words psychiatrist or "psycho" are very anxiety provoking to some men; they feel that their weaknesses are about to be exposed, and that psychiatrists have powers of reading minds. Large numbers of prisoners express greater fear and horror about mental hospitals than they do about prisons. To compensate to some extent for these difficulties, there are positive factors motivating prisoners towards co-operation, an interview sometimes means a welcome contact with the outside world even possibly finding a sympathetic ally who will suddenly set the world aright.

The selected men were collected through the normal prison medical call-up arrangements and given no information until they arrived at the interview room. Each man was told that a prison health survey was being conducted throughout England and Wales, and that he had been selected to take part in this because of his black-outs, or on a random basis as a fit man (whichever was appropriate). He was told that the survey was confidential and no information obtained would be passed on to the Home Office, the police, or any other "authority". Each man was assured that there was no obligation to co-operate.

It is gratifying that only one man refused to talk at all, and only about ten or eleven out of the 284 were noticeably obstructive and uncooperative in the interview. Most of the sessions lasted between 45 minutes and 1 hour, and only three or four lasted as long as two hours.

The interviews were semi-structured, making inquiries about the following aspects:

Occupational history for past 5 years

Past criminal history

Nature of present offence

Social background (including father's job, any parental loss, type of childhood home)

Present social situation (marital status, living conditions)

Past psychiatric history (previous hospital admissions, previous head injury, previous suicide attempts)

Alcoholic tendencies or symptoms

Current mental state

As the interview proceeded some of the details were recorded verbatim for rating at a later date, and where possible some details were immediately transformed into a predetermined code. Sometimes, the order of items on the pre-constructed sheet had to be changed and occasionally, items were omitted altogether because of the prisoner's anxieties, hostility or reticence (the commonest topic to be omitted was the family history). At some point during the session, usually towards the end, a brief neurological examination, involving the assessment of cerebral laterality, tendon reflexes, gross muscular weakness or wasting, speech, gait, and eye movements was conducted. This was done with an absolute minimum of undressing and in the course of two or three minutes.

At the end of the interview, and examination, the prisoner's permission was sought to write to hospitals, local authorities and probation departments he had previously been in contact with. In addition he was asked if he objected to his close relatives (usually a parent or sibling) being mailed. If he had no objection to this further information being collected he signed to this effect.

Relatives' Questionnaire

In an attempt to add a limited reliability check to the data collected at interview, the relatives of the men concerned were sent a standard letter and questionnaire whenever possible. If, after an interval of one month, no reply had been received (and each questionnaire was accompanied by a stamped reply envelope), then the questionnaire was sent to them again with a second standard letter and another stamped addressed envelope. No further contacts were made if this second attempt failed.

Of the 338 cases finally included in the analysis 15 out of 158 epileptic men and 26 out of 180 non-epileptic men refused to allow their families to be contacted (this difference is not statistically significant). Completed relatives' questionnaires were finally received for 106 (67%) of the epileptic men and 115 (64%) for the non-epileptics.

A very simple relatives' questionnaire was used which asked a few questions concerning the prisoner's education, work history, birth history, childhood neuroticisms, psychiatric history, epileptic history, criminal history, and family history. This was considered preferable to a long or detailed inventory which might be daunting to unsophisticated recipients. Many of the questionnaires were returned with unsolicited information of great value — either amplifying the simple answers, or giving useful addresses for further contacts or adding entirely new details. For approximately the first 50 cases the questionnaires were sent to all known living relatives — parents, siblings, wives, children, and even sometimes to close friends, but it soon became clear that the only really fruitful informants were the parent and older siblings, so these two sources were used for the remainder of the prisoners.

The completed questionnaire was compared with the interview data (and data from other sources — see below) to check its level of agreement. If it was clear from the comparison that the questionnaire markedly disagreed with case notes, criminal records, etc. then it was discarded. If however, it largely agreed with the factual information elsewhere, then the relatives' judgments were preferred to interviewee's for discrepant items. Where disagreements arose between interview and questionnaire and the reliability could not be confirmed or refuted then a 'not known' rating was made in the data.

Ancillary Information and Investigations

At the time of the interview the interviewer had each man's prison file available to him. Some of the files on the older men, and on those with shorter sentences, contained very little of value for this project. However, many of the younger individuals had psychology reports, social work reports, medical reports and probation reports included. These were read, if possible, before the interview, and collated with the other data. After the interview, the addresses of hospitals, local authorities and probation departments supplied by the prisoner were followed up with requests for reports and information. We received an excellent response from these other sources in all regions of the country. Occasionally access to information was refused on the grounds that it was too confidential for research usage, but such refusals were rare. Altogether we were able to obtain previous hospital information on 134 (85%) of the 158 epileptics and 64 (36%) of the non-epileptics, and other types of report on 97 (61%) of the epileptics and 66 (37%) of the controls.

The notes were of particular value because they sometimes contained previous medical and psychiatric diagnoses, and verbatim accounts of fits and attacks. Just occasionally considerable family details were available in the social reports.

In view of the difficulties of a nation wide survey in a non-clinical setting very few ancillary investigations were undertaken. However, the Prison Medical Department kindly agreed to help where EEG information was lacking. It proved extremely difficult to arrange many of these tests as a lot of the prisoners had only a short period to serve, and transportation to outside hospitals usually had to be arranged. However, eventually EEG information was obtained on 113 (84·2%) of the epileptic men.

Definition of Epilepsy

The diagnosis of epilepsy is a problem fraught with subjectivity and difficulty. Some would agree with Williams that "no positive definition can be applied to epilepsy because the epileptic disorder may interrupt or mimic any aspect of normal movement, feeling or thought". The Cohen Committee (Ministry of Health) also decided that "the problem of finding a formal definition is not of immediate practical importance." However, the clinician has to face this difficulty day by day in his work and arrive at decisions and categories. To make comparisons within his data the research worker cannot allow himself the luxury of diagnostic flexibility and must define his criteria, however arbitrarily, from the outset and keep them constant throughout his study. Nevertheless, this self-imposed rigidity can in itself be a snare for the criteria used in one study are often markedly different from those used in another, prohibiting inter-study comparison. Therefore, in addition to a rigid definition the researcher has to find one with which few will disagree so that later comparisons can be made with his data.

Many would agree with Symonds that very little qualification need be added to Jackson's 1890 definition: "(epilepsy is) the name for occasional, sudden, excessive, rapid and local discharges of grey matter." It is remarkable how this early definition has stood the tests of time and advancing knowledge but as Hill (1963) points out "epilepsy is not a disease but may be a symptom of many diseases" and therefore sub-classifications are essential for a meaningful diagnosis.

Most modern definitions agree with Jackson by implying something about disordered brain function from the observed clinical phenomena. For example, The College of General Practitioners in 1960 defined the epileptic attacks as "all attacks primarily cerebral in origin in which there is a disturbance of movement, feeling, behaviour, or consciousness, i.e. excluding fainting, aural vertigo, and psychologically determined attacks". Lennox and Lennox (1960) went further than this and defined epilepsy as: "a disorder of the brain expressed as paroxysmal cerebral dysrhythmia. This dysrhythmia, if symptomatic, is associated with seizures composed of one or more of the following recurrent and involuntary phenomena:

(i) loss or derangement of consciousness or remembrance (amnesia),
(ii) excess or loss of muscle tone and movement,
(iii) alteration of sensation, including hallucinations of special senses,
(iv) disturbance of the autonomic nervous system with resulting vegetative and visceral phenomena of various sorts
(v) other psychic manifestations, abnormal thought-processes or moods".

Such a definition, whilst giving guidance about clinical symptomatology leaves undefined the term "paroxysmal cerebral dysrhythmia" and would seem to include patients with EEG changes only. Hill (1963) makes his definition entirely clinical: "The more or less sudden occasion of motor, visceral, physical, or behavioural symptoms — events which in any given patient are likely to recur throughout his life as episodic phenomena, at times related to known precipitating circumstances, but not necessarily so", but he goes on to explain that "the episodic phenomena, defined by the symptoms, can only be understood in terms of excitability changes in some part or parts of the nervous system."

Many classifications of these phenomena have been used, sometimes from the clinical point of view and sometimes from the electroencephalographic. Perhaps the most widely used system, by reason of its attempt to closely relate EEG and clinical phenomena has come from the so-called "McGill Studies" which based their classification on the location of a presumed epileptic focus in the brain (Jasper and Kershman, 1941; Jasper and Kershman, 1949).

A very comprehensive classification which attempted to embrace clinical, electroencephalographic, anatomical and aetiological factors was presented by a Commission on Terminology of the International Federation of Societies for Electroencephalography and Neurophysiology in 1964 (Gastaut, et al.). However for the purposes of the present study which depended largely upon a clinical evaluation a more clinically orientated phenomenological definition and classification was formulated as follows:

EPILEPSY is said to occur in someone who has had 3 or more epileptic seizures, either during the past two years, or, if before that time, is still on regular anticonvulsant medication. AN EPILEPTIC SEIZURE is an intermittent, stereotyped disturbance of behaviour, emotion, motor function, or sensation which on clinical grounds is judged to be the result of pathological cortical neuronal discharge.

Rating Procedure

After all the relevant clinical and social data, together with any EEG reports, had been collected, a clinical extract was prepared for each case in the proband group. This extract contained the following information:

Details of any epileptic family history

Details of any history of brain damage or head trauma

The medical history relevant to epilepsy, i.e. any history of fits, blackouts, etc., giving both the patient's account and any independent accounts obtained.

A verbatim account of any fits witnessed

Recent drinking history

The anticonvulsant history

Complete EEG reports (and sometimes tracings were also attached). In the preparation of the extract full use was made of all sources of information, especially previous hospital files. The extract contained no information which could give a clue as to the patient's offence, or past criminal record.

These extracts were then rated by the author who had interviewed all but five of the men and obviously knew the full details, and by a consultant epileptologist (Dr. G. Fenton) who used only the constructed extracts. It was decided that, in the circumstances of the study, this would produce the best set of diagnostic judgments. Each rater separately rated each man as "definitely epileptic", "doubtfully epileptic", and "non-epileptic" using the definition above, erring on the cautious side and tending to rate "doubtful" or "non-epileptic" if serious doubts came into his mind.

Using this system, there were 30 out of the 192 cases in which agreement was not reached initially (15·6% disagreement).

The two raters then discussed these 30 cases individually in detail. Eventually it was possible to obtain complete agreement for the whole group.

The prison medical officers had regarded 25% of the sample as doubtfully epileptic, whereas with fuller information and a standard definition we were able to include 82% as definitely epileptic (Table 14). All the "doubtful" and "non-epileptic" cases as rated by the standardised procedure (34 in all) were omitted from the main

Table 14 **Prison Doctors' and Survey Ratings Compared**

Prison M.O. Ratings		Survey Ratings		
		Epileptic	Doubtful	Non-Ep.
Epileptic	144 (75%)	126	9	9
Doubtful	48 (25%)	32	7	9
Total	192 (100%)	158 (82%)	16 (8%)	18 (9%)

statistical analysis. Hence, for the remainder of the study, the probands appear as a group of 158.

These ratings were conducted at the end of the data collection and therefore, because of the nature of the survey, no replacement probands for the drop-outs could be obtained.

The control cases were submitted to a slightly different procedure in that all the men who gave a history of "fits", "attacks", "epilepsy", "funny turns" etc., were especially noted together with those who were subsequently (from other sources) noted to have such a history and then discussed individually, in detail, between the raters. Here the objectives were directed less towards an accurate diagnosis and more towards the exclusion of possible epileptics to ensure that the control group really did consist of non-epileptics.

Using this procedure three men were rated "doubtfully epileptic", three "definitely epileptic", one as "not known", and five as "recovered epileptics" (i.e. definite epileptics who have had no fits or medication during the past two years). This means that 12 cases were rejected from the control series leaving 180 non-epileptic prisoners for the statistical analysis. As before, the nature of the survey prevented replacement cases being obtained.

Re-examination of the One-Night Census

These figures indicate that the use of the total returns furnished by the Prison Medical Department (definite epileptics + doubtful epileptics) may have produced a slight overestimate of the prevalence of epilepsy in prisons on the one night in December 1966 (Table 12). If therefore those figures are reduced to 82% of their original value an estimated prevalence of 7·2/1000 is obtained, which is still significantly different from the 4·5/1000 obtained by the College of General Practitioners (1960) for the general population (X^2 = 32·3, 1 d.f., $p<0·0005$). Table 15 shows the original total of 271 cases referred by the Prison Medical Officers broken down in the proportions we obtained in the interview survey.

Although this figure must be taken as the most accurate estimate from the data available there are two clues that it may be an *underestimate:*

(i) Only three cases in the definite epileptics (author's ratings) were without *grand mal* seizures; this is unusual clinical experience and

could be interpreted as suggesting that some cases with auto-
matisms only have been omitted.

(ii) the control group of so-called non-epileptics revealed three cases
which fitted into the author's category of definite epilepsy, and a
further three cases of possible epilepsy.

Table 15   December Census Reclassified

Census figures for one night — December 1966		Re-rated figures
Definite Epileptics	190	223 (82%) (7·2/1000)
Doubtful Epileptics	81	23 (8%)
Non-Epileptic	—	25 (4%)
Total	271 (8·7/1000)	271 (100%)

(Total prisoners at risk = 30,993)

Types of Epilepsy

For the purpose of this study the seizures have been divided into 4
categories, on the assumption that these provide evidence of the site of
the onset of the seizure discharge. These are defined as follows:

(a) *Subcortical*

Seizures which occur in an individual who gives no account of initial
phenomena* other than generalised myoclonus and for whom there is
no clinical or EEG evidence of acquired cerebral pathology, but who
exhibits bilaterally synchronous spike and wave discharges in the EEG.

(b) *Focal Cortical — Temporal*

Seizures which occur in an individual who *either* clearly describes
sudden, stereotyped initial phenomena which he recognises as foreign
to his usual self and which can be classified under one or more of the
following categories: sensations or hallucinations of smell or taste;
complex auditory or visual hallucinations, perceptual illusions con-

---

*Initial phenomena are the beginning of an epileptic seizure irrespective of whether
they are sensory, motor, or physical, and whether or not they are followed by a major
generalised seizure (after Penfield and Kristiansen, 1951).

cerning the self, the environment or time; epigastric sensations; affective changes, mainly fear or elation; *or* shows EEG evidence of unequivocal focal spike or sharp wave discharges in one or both anterior or mid-temporal regions.

(c) *Focal Cortical — Other*

Either, (i) seizures which begin with progressive, consistently lateralised motor or sensory phenomena other than those described above, and/or accompanied by dysphasia (initial or post-ictal), and/or forced thinking, and/or simple visual hallucinations, and/or a sudden field defect *or* (ii) generalised convulsions occurring in patients with unequivocal evidence of previous cortical damage.

(d) *Unrateable*

Any epileptic seizure as defined in the primary definition which has none of the distinguishing features of the other secondary definitions. (This group mainly includes episodes of unconsciousness without initial phenomena, or without clear evidence of cortical damage, or initiated by non-specific symptoms such as giddiness, vertigo, faintness or headache).

These categories are mutually exclusive.

As before, the sheets of extracted information were used and discussions were held on points of disagreement until 100% concurrence was obtained. 15% were regarded as subcortical, 30% as temporal, 20% as other focal and 35% as unrateable (Table 16).

It is unfortunate, although perhaps inevitable when investigatory facilities are limited that the largest group should be the unrateable

Table 16   Subcategories of Epilepsy

	Nos.	Ages*	
		Mean	s.d.
Subcortical	23 (15%)	26·0	10·6
Temporal	48 (30%)	30·9	12·3
Other Focal	31 (20%)	27·1	8·9
Unrateable	56 (35%)	29·5	9·8
Total	158 (100%)	28·9	10·6

*$F = 1·5$ NS

category. Nevertheless, it is interesting to note that of the 102 cases where a definitive diagnosis was made nearly half (47%) were classified as temporal lobe cases. It will be seen from the table that no significant age variation occurred between the subgroups.

Scanty and conflicting data are available about the proportion of focal temporal lobe cases to be found in the general population of epileptics and perhaps we should own up to our ignorance by confessing with Gastaut (1953) that the nearest estimate we can make is that the frequency lies somewhere between 30 and 80% of cases! Juul-Jensen disagreed with even this wide estimate for he reported only about 24% of his cases to be "temporal lobe epilepsy", but he did show that the criminals among his outpatient series have a similar prevalence of temporal lobe cases (26%).

Matching of Probands and Controls

As we have seen the comparison group was selected with matching for sex, institution and day of admission to that institution. Prisoners are not randomly allocated after their sentences they are sent to differing regimes according to their age, sentence length, escape potential,

Table 17   Age Groupings of the Two Samples

Age Groups	Probands		Controls	
	No.	%	No.	%
15-19	34	21·5	33	18·3
20-24	34	21·5	52	28·9
25-29	29	18·4	37	20·6
30-34	20	12·7	19	10·6
35-39	14	8·9	13	7·2
40-44	10	6·3	12	6·7
45-49	9	5·7	9	5·0
50-54	4	2·5	3	1·7
55-59	3	1·9	0	0
60 +	1	0·6	2	1·1
Total	158	100	180	100
Mean:	28·9		27·7	
S.D.:	10·62		9·77	

$t = 1·11$ 336 d.f. NS

Table 18   Sentences

	Epileptics		Controls	
	No.	%	No.	%
Convicted Remands	4	3	2	1
Borstal	45	28	49	27
D.C.	0	0	0	0
0- 3 months in prison	17	11	14	8
4- 6 ,, ,,	21	13	21	12
7-12 ,, ,,	16	10	21	12
13-36 ,, ,,	33	21	41	23
3 + 10 years in prison	15	10	26	14
10 + ,, ,,	2	1	1	1
Life ,, ,,	5	3	5	3
	158	100	180	100

$X^2 = 4 \cdot 01$ (6 d.f.) NS

training needs, health requirements, and so on. Hence matching prisoners for institution will inevitably produce secondary matching in some of these other characteristics. Table 17 illustrates how closely the controls are matched with the probands in respect of age. Table 18 indicates that the expected secondary matching for sentence length is also found. It should be noted, of course that the age and sentence structure of this resident prison population are quite different (amalgamating "remanded", "10 +" and "Life", and omitting D.C.) from the reception population (Table 6). This is because older men tend to receive longer sentences, and a long sentence greatly increases an individual's chance of appearing in a resident sample.

CHAPTER 4

Criminal Characteristics

As has already been made clear we cannot determine anything about a supposed relationship between epilepsy and "crime" from a prison survey. Furthermore we have seen from the previous chapter that a comparison between the epileptics in this survey and their controls will be biased towards finding no differences because the 2 groups are matched in terms of sentence length and prison. In spite of this it is worth examining the criminal characteristics of the 2 prison samples to see just what types of crime are being committed, whether any major differences emerge between the epileptics and the non-epileptics in spite of the inbuilt bias, and how far we can explain some of the offences of the probands in purely epileptic terms.

Nature of the Offences

In prison the nature of the current offence for each man is written in his official file, and sometimes the file will also contain extracts from the police depositions or the judge's summing-up. To complete the picture for this survey each man was asked about the crime, how it happened, his part in it, his motives, and his previous criminal record. Fortunately we were able to check the prisoner's story about his past record because for the vast majority of cases either the prison concerned or the Criminal Records Office in London was kind enough to supply us with the official list of previous convictions. This official list usually only noted indictable offences.

One of the striking things about the interviews was the frankness of the men concerned; very few refused to talk about their current offence, and although many minor errors were made by the men reporting their past offences it was a rarity to come across a case which showed gross distortion of the information. If anything, prisoners recounted more offences than the C.R.O. did. Any omissions were included in the data if the remainder of the interview was deemed reliable and the prisoner's account of his record was otherwise accurate.

The present offences and the previous offences were grouped into three broad categories:

(a) Property offence, which included obtaining money by false pretences, falsification of accounts, fraudulent conversion, embezzlement, forgery, counterfeiting, larceny, receiving, taking and driving away, housebreaking, office breaking, warehouse breaking, shopbreaking, burglary, demanding money by menaces, possessing housebreaking implements.

(b) Violence offences, which included common assault, actual bodily harm, robbery, grievous bodily harm, cruelty to children, murder, manslaughter, culpable homicide.

(c) Sex offences which included buggery, indecency, rape, indecent assault, unlawful sexual intercourse, incest, living on the earnings of a prostitute, indecent exposure.

It will be noticed that many non-indictable offences such as motoring offences, loitering, vagrancy, railway offences, begging, and threatening behaviour have been omitted. These were excluded because such offences are quoted inconsistently in the official criminal records. However, it is possible for an individual to be imprisoned for this type of offence, and when this had occurred for a subject's *current* offence it was assigned to a separate 'other' group. If two or more charges were preferred simultaneously then the most serious offence was the one counted (seriousness being measured in terms of punishment given or if the offences were punished equally, it was measured in terms of a simple seriousness scale: homicide, violence, arson, rape, sex, fraud, larceny, drugs, drink, other).

Table 19 demonstrates that the epileptics committed the same types of offences as their controls. We cannot draw a conclusion from this as it may well be a secondary matching effect. It should be noted that 6 of the epileptics were convicted of homicide, a clinical experience in marked contrast to that of Lennox who has already been quoted as saying that "over a period of 35 years I remember only 2 instances of murder by epileptics" (Lennox and Lennox, Vol. 2) or that of Älstrom who found in his large clinic sample no cases of serious aggression, manslaughter or murder. This striking difference serves to re-emphasise that different observers using different viewpoints and different sampling procedures see different things. It would be quite wrong to argue from the experience of Älstrom or Lennox that epileptics don't commit seriously aggressive crimes, or from this data that 4% of epileptic criminals are murderers because each observer is using a selected sample and then commenting upon one of the selection criteria.

Table 19   Current Offences

	Epileptics		Controls	
	No.	%	No.	%
Property	105	66	108	60
Violent*	23	15	40	22
Sex	14	9	12	7
Other	16	10	20	11
Total	158	100	180	100

$X^2 = 3.81$ (3 d.f.) NS

*This includes 6 epileptics and 4 controls convicted of homicide (murder or manslaughter)

Examination of the 6 epileptic homicide cases in this series shows that there is nothing unusual in the circumstances of the offence. None of the prisoners claimed amnesia for the attack, all but one were the result of rage reactions and directed towards a family member or lover. The one exception showed some evidence of premeditation but stated that the murderous feelings suddenly came over him in an argument with the victim and that the premeditated plans were completely forgotten. Only one man had ever been previously convicted of a violent offence, two were virtually first offenders. Two of the control cases were also first offenders. Three of them had killed their wives or girlfriends but this group included a man who had murdered in the course of burglary.

An interesting and possibly important feature discernible with the epileptic group is shown in Table 20 where it will be seen that when the two main groups of offenders (property offenders and violent offenders) are examined in relation to the subtypes of epilepsy there are no significant differences in distribution. It will be remembered (from p. 43). that the subgroups do not differ in terms of age.

Table 20 **Property and violent offenders by epileptic diagnosis**

| | Property | | Violence | | Total |
	No.	%	No.	%	N
Subcortical	15	79	4	21	19 (100%)
Temporal	34	83	7	17	41 (100%)
Other focal	22	82	5	19	27 (100%)
Unrateable	34	83	7	17	41 (100%)
Total	105		23		

$X^2 = 0.17$ (3 d.f.) NS

Degree of Violence

One drawback in using the rather arbitrary classification of the offences given above is that sometimes the legal description is a matter of chance; for example if two men fight in a public house, injuries received by one or other of the men may well depend upon such chance factors as weapons available, the exact site of impact, the intervention of other people, etc. It is possible for example for a serious attempt to injure or kill someone to misfire and be classified as an "assault" whilst a man only marginally involved in a bank hold-up will probably be charged with robbery with violence.

A method was devised for roughly assessing the degree of violence involved in each offence. All the details that could be gleaned about each offence were gathered from the prisoner's own description, the prison notes, any police or court material available, and occasionally from press cuttings. This was then typed on to a single sheet of paper which had no reference to other factors in the prisoner's history and was given entirely blind to two raters who had not interviewed the man and who each independently attempted to assign the crime to the following four-point violence scale.

0 — *No violence*

1 — *Violence to Property* — a violent act using physical force in a destructive manner towards an inanimate object or an animal, with evidence of disturbed mood.

2 — *Moderate Violence to a Person* — a violent act using, threatening, or being involved in the use of, physical force towards another person, and yet not amounting to severe violence.

3 — *Severe Violence to a Person* — a violent act using physical force against another person damaging or seriously endangering their life or health.

9 — *Unrateable* — (this excludes doubts between categories when the higher rating is used)

N.B. (Rating 1 includes the criterion of "disturbed mood" in an attempt to exclude housebreakers and others who damage property in the course of theft — their prime objective.)

When each rater had classified each of the 338 crimes committed by the prisoners they were examined for agreement. At this initial stage the raters disagreed in only 47 cases (13·2 per cent disagreement). They were then given these cases to reconsider, knowing that the other rater had come to a different conclusion about them but without knowing in which direction they differed. After such reconsideration only 16 cases (5 epileptics and 11 controls) were the source of disagreement (4·2 per cent disagreement). These 16 cases were added to the unrateable category.

A cross-tabulation of the degree of violence with the type of offence (Table 21) shows that there was a pronounced agreement between the category of offence as applied by the court and the violence rating given in the survey.

Table 21   **Degree of violence cross-tabulated with official categories of offence (epileptics and controls together)**

	Property	Violence	Sex	Other	Total
Violence 0	209	1	16	23	249
Violence 1	4	0	0	2	6
Violence 2	4	23	1	1	29
Violence 3	1	28	0	0	29
Total	218	52	17	26	313

(25 cases were 'violence unrateable')

Table 20 has demonstrated that there were no significant differences between the epileptics and the controls in terms of the official categories used, and in view of the close similarity between the official and the independent rating system used here we can expect little or no difference between the groups in terms of the degree of violence. Table 22 confirms that this is the case.

Table 23 shows that the presence of violence in the present offence is unrelated to the diagnostic subtype for the epileptic group.

Table 22   Degrees of violence compared (epileptics v. controls)

	Epileptics	Controls
Violence 0	123 (82%)	124 (77%)
Violence 1	3	5
Violence 2	10	19
Violence 3	15	14
Total	151	162

X^2 = 2·93 (2 d.f.) NS (amalgamating violence 1 and violence 2) (7 epileptics and 18 controls were 'violence unrateable')

Table 23   Epileptic diagnosis and degree of violence

	Degree of Violence				
	0		1, 2 & 3		
	N	%	N	%	Total
Subcortical	17	81	4	19	21 (100%)
Temporal	36	78	10	22	46 (100%)
Other focal	25	81	6	19	31 (100%)
Unrateable	45	85	8	15	53 (100%)
Total	123		28		151

X^2 = 0·59 (2 d.f.) NS
(amalgamating 'subcortical' and 'unrateable')
(7 cases were 'violence unrateable')

Previous Offences

Each man's previous offences were categorised in the same way as his current offences. The number of convictions officially recorded were supplemented by the prisoner's account of his juvenile convictions, but non indictable offences (e.g. motoring offences, malicious damage, drunkenness, loitering, poaching) were excluded. Charges taken into consideration or offences dealt with at the same court session were not counted as extra convictions. If 2 or more convictions occurred simultaneously then the most serious was the one counted, seriousness being measured in terms of punishment given or in terms of punishment potential.

Table 24 reveals that overall the groups are well matched for the

Table 24 Previous convictions compared between the groups

No. of Pre cons	Property		Violence		Sexual		Total	
	Eps	Controls	Eps	Controls	Eps	Controls	Eps	Controls
0	14 (9%)	20 (11%)	114 (73%)	127 (72%)	133 (85%)	159 (90%)	9 (6%)	13 (7%)
1	20	12	19	26	14	10	14	11
2	21	19	14	17	4	5	18	14
3-9	72	103	9	7	5	3	79	103
10+	29 (19%)	23 (13%)	0	0	0	0	36 (23%)	36 (20%)
Total*	156	177	156	177	156	177	156	177
Mean no. of pre cons	5·25	5·11	0·53	0·48	0·30	0·16	6·23	6·20
S.D.	4·58	4·20	—	—	—	—	4·99	4·58
t-test (331 d.f.)	0·28 NS		0·134 NS		1·38 NS		0·06 NS	

N.B. For violent and sexual offences log x + 1 has been used as the variate.
*2 epileptics and 3 control cases have been omitted from this comparison as the relevant data could not be obtained.

total number of previous convictions they have incurred, furthermore, there is no significant difference between the epileptics and controls in the number of previous convictions for violence.

On the other hand Table 25 indicates that the different diagnostic subgroups within the epileptic groups have different patterns of criminality. The temporal lobe cases have more previous convictions overall, but it is the subcortical cases who have accumulated a disproportionately large share of the violent convictions, and the 'other focal' cases a disproportionately small share. Once again it should be noted that the subgroups do not differ in terms of age.

Table 25 Epileptic subgroups compared for number and type of previous convictions

No. of previous convictions	Subcortical $n = 22$		Temporal $n = 47$		Other focal $n = 31$		Unrateable $n = 56$		Total $n = 156$	
	N	C	N	C	N	C	N	C	N	C
Violent	18	0·82	25	0·53	7	0·23	29	0·52	79	0·51
Non-violent	82	3·73	326	6·94	167	5·39	302	5·39	877	5·62
Total	100	4·55	351	7·47	174	5·61	331	5·91	956	6·13

C = number of previous convictions per case
Overall $x^2 = 17·34$ (3 d.f.) $p<0·001$
Other focal v. rest $x^2 = 5·05$ (1 d.f.) $p<0·05$
Subcort. v. rest $x^2 = 13·97$ (1 d.f.) $p<0·0005$
Total temp v. total rest $t = 20·54$ (154 d.f.) $p<0·001$
(using log $x + 1$ as the variate)

Automatism

Perhaps much of the sustained interest in epilepsy as a criminological problem is due to the reputed association between the phenomenon of automatism which occurs in epilepsy and some apparently motiveless crimes. Most textbooks of forensic psychiatry urge us to consider automatism as a possible defence in violent offences; for example, Maudsley (1906) remarked that "if it (the deed) has been done with great violence, without indications of premeditation, without apparent motive, and without secrecy, and if the accused person is discovered to be the victim of epilepsy, it is possible that it has been done in a paroxysm following an epileptic fit". In his textbook East (1927) devoted a whole chapter to the features one should look for it consider-ing this defence. He regarded a previous history of epilepsy as crucial. Next he pointed out that some emphasised that behaviour could only be considered as an automatism if it was stereotyped; but he warned that there may be exceptions to this rule. His final two criteria were that the act should be a caricature of normal behaviour and that amnesia for the act should usually be present. As an appendix to his chapter he cited 6 illustrative cases, some of which do not satisfactorily fit even his own criteria of epileptic automatism.

The first strangled his pregnant wife during sexual intercourse, attempted suicide after the event, and claimed amnesia for the homicide. A feeble-minded man of 45 years removed a baby from its pram and nursed it for a few minutes against its mother's wishes. Two other cases were suicidal attempts in depressed patients and the question of amnesia was not raised. The fifth patient made several unprovoked dangerous assaults on his wife and landlady but re-membered the events. The final one concerned a struggle involving two policemen and an ambulance man with a patient who had some minutes previously been seen to have a fit in the street.

In his textbook "Psychiatry and the Criminal", MacDonald (1969) points out that, despite the considerable medicolegal interest in epilepsy, "authors are seldom able to quote a case from their own experience and the few case reports available are copied from one textbook to another." MacDonald, in a personal series of over 1000 court reports, could recall only two examples of crimes committed as a result of an epileptic seizure—one patient, while driving her car in a confused state following a seizure, ran over a schoolboy; the other, a youth with well-documented psychomotor attacks, killed an elderly lady.

Automatic phenomena have been systematically evaluated by Knox. He reviewed 434 epileptics attending one clinic and found in the records comments on 64 of these suggesting the presence of episodes of automatic behaviour. 43 patients were finally assessed as having such episodes which he defined as "a condition of impaired awareness in which an individual may perform an act or series of actions of a complex kind, the degree of awareness varying insofar as there may subsequently be complete amnesia for the incident or, if it can be recalled, recollection is imprecise and partial", and which were confirmed by witnesses. Seven main conclusions were drawn:

(1) Acts of violence are unusual (only one case was evident in his series).

(2) The abnormal activity tends to appear suddenly and there should be no evidence of planning.

(3) Automatic behaviour is of brief duration—minutes only.

(4) There will probably be no attempt to conceal acts undertaken during automatism.

(5) There will be no amnesia for events occurring prior to loss of consciousness.

(6) There does not necessarily need to be a history of automatism associated with previous epileptic fits.

(7) A normal EEG does not exclude the possibility of automatism.

Whilst conclusions (1) and (4) seem unjustified from his data, since he was studying a clinic population (violent automata would probably cause the patient to fall into the hands of the law, and similarly there is no need for non-law-breaking epileptics to cover the tracks of their automatic episodes), this is a reasonably objective description of the syndrome.

To investigate the possibility of automatic criminal behaviour in this survey each man was asked if he had suffered a fit within the 12 hours before or the 12 hours after the offence. Only 10 reported such fits; four said they had one just before the offence, five said just after and one man claimed both. The clinical details of these cases have been published elsewhere (Gunn and Fenton, 1971).

Very little direct or "automatic" relationship between the crimes committed and the men's epilepsy could be discerned. One man hit out at a policeman after he had been drinking and had had a fit; it was just possible that he was in a state of post-ictal confusion. Another stole some goods from a car after he had had a fit. Again the possibility of post-ictal confusion arises, especially as he took the goods back to the police station the next day. Two cases of serious violence (manslaughter, rape) seemed to be rage reactions to frustration. One man set fire to a building, allegedly in response to instructions from a hallucinatory voice, but as he was a chronic alcoholic as well as an epileptic it is difficult to attribute the hallucinations to the epilepsy alone. It is perhaps significant that none of the men claimed amnesia for his offence.

An opportunity to compare these findings with data from a Special Hospital arose because Dr G. Fenton, an adviser to this survey, examined all patients with a diagnosis of epilepsy who were in Broadmoor Hospital on January 1, 1966. Routine waking and sleep sphenoidal EEG recordings were carried out on every subject who had previously been diagnosed as suffering from epilepsy. The total number of male patients was 46. Of this group, four were excluded on the ground that they did not have clinical epilepsy; five had had a few epileptic attacks in childhood but had been free from epilepsy since then; and five were chronic schizophrenic patients, who had had isolated seizures during their psychotic illness. The remaining 32 suffered from recurrent epileptic attacks in adult life. Of this group, using the criteria previously described 17 were regarded as having temporal-lobe epilepsy, eight focal epilepsy (the focal involvement being in areas other than the temporal lobe), and 1 subcortical epilepsy; six were rated as unknown or unrateable. Using the criteria of Älstrom, ten had a known cause, 18 had a presumed known cause, and four no known cause.

The prevalence of epilepsy in Broadmoor Hospital on January 1, 1966, was thus 5%. Of the 32 men with recurrent seizures, 29 were admitted to hospital as the result of criminal offences (15 violence against the person or property, 13 homicide, and 1 other), the remaining three being transferred from conventional mental hospitals under section 26 of the 1959 Mental Health Act because of dangerously aggressive or persistently antisocial behaviour.

In the 29 who had committed offences, the relation between their behaviour at the time of the offence and the occurrence of epileptic seizures of any kind was investigated. Information was obtained by interviewing the men themselves and by studying the police reports, prison medical officers' court reports, and the Broadmoor Hospital case-notes.

Only three patients were found to have had a definite epileptic seizure within twelve hours before or after the offence leading to their admission to Broadmoor Hospital. Again the clinical details have been reported elsewhere (Gunn and Fenton).

Of these three, two men probably did commit dangerous offences in a state of altered consciousness. The first struck out during an epileptic fit at some friends he was visiting and an elderly man died. The second developed a fit after an evening shooting pigeons; the following morning, still in a state of confusion, he rose early, took his shotgun and brandished it in the village street, firing shots occasionally; fortunately nobody was killed.

The important aspects of this enquiry into "automatic" criminal behaviour in epileptics stand out:
   (i) they are very rare indeed, a survey of all English prisons and one English Special Hospital produced only one example of criminal behaviour occurring during an epileptic fit.

(ii) there is a slight possibility that some odd behaviour occurring in a post-ictal confusional phase may be mistaken for criminal behaviour.

Discussion

Plainly this survey cannot tell us about any special relationship between crime in general and epilepsy — a court survey would be needed for that; neither can it entirely settle the long dispute concerning the presence or absence of an association between epilepsy and violence. The main finding demonstrates that, as predicted, the initial matching for prison has produced secondary matching for offending. It is worth noting again, however, that the vast majority of epileptic prisoners are non-violent thieves.

It is widely believed that there is a special relationship between temporal lobe epilepsy and aggressiveness and so the intra-epileptic-group comparisons of criminality in different diagnostic sub-types are of particular interest. Interestingly, the results indicated that, whilst the temporal lobe cases had a higher previous conviction rate than the other groups, they were not specially prone to be convicted of a violent offence. This finding has to be put in the context that the group described here consisted of epileptic prisoners and not epileptic offenders in general (violent temporal lobe cases may be differentially sent to hospital), and that the group probably under-represents the true proportion of temporal lobe cases in prison. The relationship between temporal lobe epilepsy and psychiatric abnormality will be discussed at the end of Chapter 5.

The finding that it is the subcortical cases who are sentenced for disproportionately more violent offences and that the 'other focal' cases are sentenced for disproportionately fewer violent convictions is even more unexpected. The result cannot be interpreted simply in terms of years at risk (subcortical being more likely to have early onset epilepsy and 'other focal' late onset) because it is the temporal lobe group who have received a greater number of previous convictions and the finding here concerns the proportion of violent offences. It would be premature to draw the firm conclusion that it is the 'subcortical' epileptic who gets himself especially frequently into fights, etc. The finding needs confirmation from other studies, especially court studies, because once again it is possible that courts take a different attitude towards violent focal epileptics than to those with subcortical epilepsy.

Automatic behaviour seems to be a rare explanation for the crimes of epileptic patients. Post-ictal confusion may occur in some cases but it is not common. Certainly it seems unreasonable to explain the excess prevalence of epilepsy in the prisons in terms of automatic or confusional behaviour.

CHAPTER 5

Illness Factors

Mental State and Suicidal Ideas

Many previous workers have suggested a relationship between epilepsy and psychiatric abnormality. Hill (1953 and 1959) has reviewed the main psychiatric disorders of epilepsy. He concludes that personality disorder with its attendant irritability, suspiciousness, and tension is particularly likely to be seen in the temporal lobe epileptic, and that in these patients hysterical, depressive and anxiety states, usually transient in nature, are common. Hill also mentions psychotic states occurring in epileptics, this has been amplified by Pond (1957) and studied by Beard and Slater (1962) who suggested a relationship between epilepsy, particularly temporal lobe epilepsy, and schizophrenia-like psychotic states.

The incidence of psychiatric disturbance in epileptic patients is hard to determine with precision because of sampling difficulties. Pond and Bidwell (1960) found in their English general practice sample that 70 out of 245 cases (29%) showed psychological difficulties (neurosis, behaviour problems in children, "epileptic personalities", organic syndromes, alcoholism, and inadequacy of personality). Of the 39 temporal lobe cases in Pond and Bidwell's series 20 (51%) had psychological difficulties of this nature. Graham and Rutter (1968) studied the total population of 11,865 children aged 5-14 years on the Isle of Wight and found that whilst the prevalence of psychiatric disorder (neurotic disorder, anti-social disorders, mixed disorder, hyperkinetic syndrome) amongst the whole population was of the order of 6·6%, 58·3% of those with epilepsy and a lesion above the brain stem suffered from psychiatric disorder. Of the 8 children with psychomotor epilepsy 6 showed this kind of disorder and the authors comment on this strikingly high rate which is significantly above that found for other types of epilepsy.

Clinically, epilepsy also seems to be related to suicidal behaviour, and one or two studies support this contention. Prudhomme (1941) found death by suicide to be frequent amongst epileptics in New York — 67 deaths among 75,000 unclassified epileptics, and at one colony where detailed figures were available he found 1 suicide/4378 patients/ year which he estimated to be twice the mean rate found in the general population at the time, five times the mean rate if the figures were corrected for age. Delay *et al.* (1957) draw our attention to the difficulties of distinguishing between true suicide, self-mutilation and accidental death in the epileptic. Even so looking at attempted, rather than completed, suicide they estimated that of their series of 347 epileptic patients about one third made one or more suicidal attempts. This figure was confirmed by Barande (1958) who studied 94 epileptics in a prison and contrasted them with 65 in a mental hospital and also found that overall about one third of epileptics had made suicidal attempts. More recently Krohn (1963) has reported 3 suicides amongst 107 institutionalised epileptics in Norway (2·8%) and Taylor and Falconer (1968) lost five patients by suicide from 100 post temporal lobectomy epileptic patients at the end of their follow-up period (2-12 years). Henriksen *et al.* (1970) have studied the death certificates of all adult patients with the diagnosis of epilepsy discharged from four neurological clinics in Denmark. Of the 2,763 patients included 164 died during a 25 year follow up period, 60 patients from tumours, but of the remaining 104 patients 21 died by their own hand. This was against a calculated expected total of 7. Their average age at death was 32 years.

All the prisoners in this survey were given a brief mental state examination and gross neurological evaluation. Time did not allow for detailed work but an estimate was made of (i) significant mental state abnormalities, (ii) previous suicidal behaviour, (iii) significant neurological abnormalities.

Psychiatric Examination

For mental state assessments Schneider's criteria (1958) were used to diagnose schizophrenia (i.e. at least one Schneider first rank symptom had to be present for the diagnosis to be made) and the following arbitrary scales were used for depression and anxiety:

(i) depressive symptoms
Feelings of sadness or misery
Pathological guilt or self blame
Suicidal ideas
Retardation
Frequent weeping
Insomnia
Loss of appetite
Agitation
Delusions of serious illness
Despair

If 3 or 4 of these symptoms were considered present the illness was designated mild depression, if 5 or more then severe depression.

(ii) anxiety symptoms
Excess worrying
Frequent subjective tension or fear
Restlessness in interview
Badly bitten nails
Phobias
Depersonalisation feelings
*Somatic anxiety symptoms
Panic attacks

Two or three of these symptoms constituted mild anxiety whilst 4 or more were taken as indicators of severe anxiety.

For some purposes the epileptic group was divided into the clinical sub-categories, previously described, "temporal", "other-focal", and "sub-cortical". Clearly there was no possibility of direct pathological examination for each case, but the historical data were supplemented by EEG material for 113 cases (84·2%).

Each man was also asked as part of his history whether or not he had ever made a suicidal attempt and, if so, how many attempts he had made. A certain degree of reticence was encountered in this area although in those cases where a check could be made from old records, no outstanding anomalies were uncovered.

---

*Somatic anxiety symptoms included such things as palpitations, complaints of sweating, frequency of micturation, breathlessness etc. which were not considered to have organic pathology as a basis.

Psychiatric Symptoms

When examined by this means the two groups (epileptic and non-epileptic) show striking differences (Table 26). The epileptics clearly suffered more frequently from affective symptoms than did the controls. Nevertheless, the controls also showed high levels of mental abnormality which will not surprise those who work in close contact with the prison population. In view of the nature of the sample, however, this finding must not be generalised.

Table 26   Epileptics and Controls Compared for Mental State

	Epileptics	Controls
Normal	68 (43%)	106 (59%)
Mild Anxiety	20 (13%)	17 (9%)
Mild Depression	19 (12%)	29 (16%)
Moderate Anxiety	12 (8%)	8 (4%)
Moderate Depression	34 (22%)	19 (11%)
Schizophrenia	0	0
Other	5 (3%)	1 (1%)
Total	158 (100%)	180 (100%)

$X^2 = 13.72$ (4 d.f.) $p < 0.025$ (omitting Schizophrenia and other)

When the two major age groups, under 25 and over 25 are examined separately (Table 27) then we find that although the older epileptics do not differ significantly from the younger epileptics the former do differ significantly from their equivalent controls whereas the latter do not.

Table 27   Age and Mental State

Mental State	15-24 years		25 years +	
	Epileptics	Controls	Epileptics	Controls
Normal	32 (47%)	46 (55%)	36 (42%)	60 (63%)
Anxiety State	12 (18%)	11 (13%)	20 (24%)	14 (15%)
Depression	24 (35%)	27 (32%)	29 (34%)	21 (22%)
Total	68 (100%)	84 (100%)	85 (100%)	95 (100%)

$X^2 = 1.06$ (2 d.f.) NS $X^2 = 7.81$ (2 d.f.) $p < 0.025$

(Cases diagnosed as "other" abnormal mental state have been omitted.)
Between older and younger epileptics $X^2 = 0.25$ (2 d.f.) NS

The small group of "other" types of mental abnormality apart from depression, anxiety and schizophrenia are of considerable interest for of the five epileptic cases four can be considered as having brain damage, particularly frontal lobe brain damage. The fifth man, aged 27, had no known cerebral damage or disease although for many years he had been considered mentally defective and spent most of his childhood in mental deficiency colonies. However, he had always refused formal IQ tests (for elaborate paranoid reasons) and he could certainly write. His mental state was difficult to label exactly although it was clearly abnormal and showed a mixture of suspicion, hostility, euphoria and disinterestedness together with complaints of filthy thoughts pushing their way into his head and a compulsion to think things over and over again.

One possible explanation for the excess of symptoms in the epileptic group is their medication (although as both phenobarbitone and phenytoin have sedative effects, one could also reasonably hypothesise that patients on such drugs should have *less* symptoms). Only 18 of the probands were not receiving anticonvulsants and as Table 28 shows they reported proportionally more affective symptoms than patients on anticonvulsants. Although this difference does not reach statistical significance it suggests that the taking of anticonvulsive drugs is unlikely to account for the increased number of symptoms in the epileptic group.

Table 28 Mental State and Anticonvulsant Treatment

Mental State	Anticonvulsants	
	Yes	No
Normal	63 (47%)	5 (28%)
Anxiety symptoms	27 (20%)	5 (28%)
Depressive symptoms	45 (33%)	8 (44%)
Total	135 (100%)	18 (100%)

$$X^2 = 2\cdot30 \ (1 \ \text{d.f.}) \ p<0\cdot1$$
(comparing normal and abnormal)
(5 cases diagnosed as "other" abnormal mental states have been omitted.)

Cross tabulations of mental state with the degree of violence exhibited in the current offence produced categories too small for statistical analysis.

When the 4 diagnostic sub-groups of epileptics were compared for mental state abnormalities, there were no significant differences between them.

Table 29   Epileptic Diagnosis and Mental State

Type of Epilepsy	Normal	Affective Symptoms	Total
Subcortical	14 (61%)	9 (39%)	23 (100%)
Temporal	22 (47%)	25 (53%)	47 (100%)
Focal Other	13 (46%)	15 (54%)	28 (100%)
Unrateable	19 (35%)	36 (65%)	55 (100%)
Total	68 (44%)	85 (56%)	153 (100%)

$X^2 = 4.85$ (3 d.f.) NS

(5 cases diagnosed as "other" abnormal mental states have been omitted.)

Suicidal Symptoms

Table 30 shows a significant difference between the groups when compared for the presence of suicidal feelings at interview. Although not many of either group confessed to such ideas at interview, over three times as many epileptics did as controls.

Table 30   Suicidal Ideas amongst Epileptics and Controls

Suicidal Ideas	Epileptics	Controls
Absent	140 (88.6%)	174 (96.7%)
Present	18 (11.4%)	6 (3.3%)
Total	158 (100%)	180 (100%)

$X^2 = 8.29$ (1 d.f.) $p < 0.005$

Again, it is possible to suggest that this difference in mental state is attributable to the depressant effect of the anticonvulsant which the probands were receiving. However, when the 18 without anticonvulsants are compared with the remainder they clearly have a very similar proportion with suicidal ideas. Age, employment, criminal factors and type of epilepsy were found to be unrelated to suicidal ideas at interview. Not surprisingly, the number of suicide attempts made in the past correlated significantly and positively with the presence of suicidal ideas at interview ($r = 0·327$ for the probands, $n = 154$, $p<0·001$ and $r = 0·496$ for the controls, $n = 177$, $p<0·001$). This finding, taken in conjunction with the difference between the groups for suicidal ideas leads to the expectation of more previous suicidal attempts being made among the epileptics than the controls. Table 31 clearly demonstrates that this is so.

Table 31   Suicide Attempts

	Epileptics	Controls
Previous suicide attempt	60 (39%)	39 (22%)
No previous suicide attempt	94 (61%)	138 (78%)
Total	154 (100%)	177 (100%)

$X^2 = 11·7$ (1 d.f.) $p<0·001$

(Data were missing for 3 controls and 4 epileptic cases.)

However, there are no significant differences between the groups when the age at which the first suicide attempt was made is considered. Like the data for suicidal ideas when correlations between actual suicidal attempts and the other integral variables are made no relationships were found.

Interestingly, there was a relationship between the epileptic diagnostic category and previous suicidal behaviour, the temporal lobe epileptics and the undiagnosable group being more likely to have suffered a suicidal incident.

Table 32   Epileptic Subcategories and Suicidal Behaviour

	Subcortical	Temporal	Other Focal	N/K	Total
Previous suicide attempt	5 (21·7%)	25 (52·1%)	7 (23·3%)	23 (43·4%)	60 (39%)
No previous suicide attempt	18 (78·3%)	23 (47·9%)	23 (76·7%)	30 (56·6%)	94 (61%)
Total	23 (100%)	48 (100%)	30 (100%)	53 (100%)	154 (100%)

$X^2 = 9·86$ (3 d.f.) $p<0·025$

(Data were missing for 4 epileptic cases.)

Drinking Problems

For two important reasons it was considered essential to examine the extent and nature of the drinking problems which this population exhibits. Firstly it is well known that alcohol drinking is of considerable criminological significance; e.g. Banay (1942) found that 45% of the men admitted to Sing Sing prison were alcoholics and showed that there was a special association between alcoholism and offences against the person. Gibbens and Silberman (1970) record that of 404 short term prisoners in London 22% had a previous drunkenness conviction and another 18% (40% in all) had drinking behaviour which seriously interfered with their social adjustment, and furthermore the heavy drinkers had more than the expected proportion of aggressive offences. Edwards *et al.* (1971) reported alcoholism to vary among prisoners between 11% and 60%. Secondly alcoholism is important because there is a known association between epilepsy and alcohol. Lees (1967) maintains that any form of epilepsy may be precipitated by alcohol in those who already have the susceptibility. Withdrawal of alcohol from an addict can precipitate seizures (Isbell *et al.*, 1955; Victor and Adams, 1953; Victor and Brausch, 1967) and a number of cerebral degenerative disorders have been associated with excessive drinking and these can no doubt produce in their turn symptomatic epileptic fits (Lees, 1967). Clearly then a high association between criminality and alcohol, and between alcohol and epilepsy, makes the interpretation of a survey of epileptic criminals more complicated.

To reinforce these points and indicate the clinical dilemmas that can arise, one or two cases from the survey are worth quoting:

"Alfred", who suffered from a frontal lobe syndrome, had clear evidence of cerebral atrophy, and his resting EEG showed diffuse abnormalities; in addition he suffered from *grand mal* seizures and was a chronic skid row alcoholic. His own observation was that alcohol precipitates the fits. Although he came within the definition of "epileptic" used in this survey clearly in this example alcoholism and epilepsy are inextricably mixed. Conversely, "Brian" an alcoholic who has had many withdrawal symptoms over the past few years but had started to suffer with "blackouts", i.e. losses of consciousness, during the two months before his imprisonment, one at least probably accompanied by seizure-like activity, was not considered to be epileptic. "Colin" a man of 26 years, killed a man whilst he was under the influence of a large dose of alcohol. For many years he had been a heavy weekend rum drinker and had even suffered the occasional morning shakes and amnesia attacks as a result of this. His epilepsy started at 7 with *petit mal* seizures and later developed into infrequent *grand mal* seizures, for which he has received regular phenytoin medication for some years. After the offence EEG studies showed that resting patterns were disturbed by theta activity of moderate amplitude, but after ingestion of alcohol a host of abnormalities appeared, especially spike and wave delta and theta activity. His conviction was reduced from murder to culpable homicide by reason of diminished responsibility. Again, the man presented a complex picture with the strong possibility that if his drinking had stopped so might his seizures. Nevertheless, he fell within the defined criteria and he has been included as an epileptic. In contra-distinction, however, there are other cases like "David" also convicted of homicide. He killed a casual girl-friend whilst drunk and whilst having intercourse with her. He, too, was an alcoholic and suffered from various alcoholic symptoms including "blackouts" but there is no clear record of anything resembling a seizure and when his EEG was recorded under the provocation of alcohol, abnormalities were noted but nothing specifically epileptic. His conviction was not reduced from murder and he appeared in the control group as non-epileptic.

In view of the intermingling of the pathological processes present in both epilepsy and alcoholism it is obviously important to determine in what ways the epileptic group differs from the control group in respect of drinking habits and complications.

For the purpose of the present study six measures of the severity of drinking and its complications were obtained from the history elicited at interview. Firstly, each man was asked about the extent of his drinking and this was rated on the following 3 point frequency scale:

0 = Abstainer or very rarely drinks

1 = Moderate drinker, e.g. weekends only, or once or twice per week

2 = Heavy drinker—a man who drinks regularly every day or to intoxication at frequent intervals

Next, five questions were asked about previous symptoms likely to be due to alcoholic addiction and these were each rated 0 if the patient denied ever having them or admitted to them on one occasion only, and 1 if he recalled them for at least two occasions in the past.

(a) Attacks of amnesia—total loss of memory for a circumscribed period of time associated with heavy drinking.

(b) Tremors—gross shaking of two or more limbs made worse by intention following a heavy drinking episode.

(c) Hallucinations, auditory or visual in association with heavy drinking.

(d) Morning drinking—resorting to alcohol soon after waking to relieve the effects of a previous drinking episode.

(e) Crude spirit drinking—indulgence in cheap spirits not intended for internal consumption such as methylated spirit, surgical spirit, eau de cologne etc.

Alcoholic Symptoms

Examination of the overall between-group differences (Tables 33 and 34) shows remarkably little distinction. The only difference between the groups is that the epileptics drank less moderately than the controls ($X^2 = 5\cdot13$, 1 d.f., $p<0\cdot025$), i.e. they drank very much less or very much more than the controls.

Table 33   Drinking Frequency

	Abstainers and rare drinkers	Moderate drinkers	Heavy drinkers	Total
Epileptics	38 (25%)	44 (28%)	73 (47%)	155 (100%)
Controls	33 (18%)	72 (40%)	74 (41%)	179 (100%)

(Data were missing for 3 epileptics and 1 control.)

$X^2 = 5\cdot42$ (2 d.f.) NS

Table 34   Alcoholic symptoms

	Epileptics	Controls	X^2 (1 d.f.)
Amnesia attacks	38 (25%)	45 (25%)	0·003 NS
Alcoholic tremors	28 (18%)	39 (22%)	0·490 NS
Hallucinations	13 (8%)	9 (5%)	1·688 NS
Morning drinking	35 (23%)	35 (20%)	0·595 NS
Crude spirit drinking	4 (3%)	5 (3%)	0·010 NS
Total rated	155	179	

(Data were missing for 3 epileptics and 1 control.)
(It should be noted that the symptoms are not mutually exclusive.)

Alcoholic Diagnosis

Isolating separate features of the phenomenology of heavy drinking behaviour in this way is useful for a detailed examination but the clinician tends to diagnose "alcoholism" as an all or none phenomenon. Presumably he makes a mental addition of such factors as the ones isolated here and uses a personal arbitrary criterion for the presence or absence of the condition. If the present data is examined by counting any individual who admits to three or more of the features shown in Table 34 as suffering from alcoholism we find that again the probands and controls are closely matched (Table 35).

Table 35   Patients diagnosed as alcoholics in terms of 3 or more alcoholic symptoms

	Alcoholics	Others	Total
Epileptics	26 (16·8%)	129 (83·2%)	155 (100%)
Controls	27 (15·1%)	152 (84·9%)	179 (100%)

(Data were missing for 3 epileptics and 1 control.)

If we now examine the four subgroups distinguished in Table 35 in terms of their variation on other factors we find that the control alcoholics started their criminal careers much later than the other groups and the epileptic alcoholics have made more suicidal attempts (Table 36). There is also a trend for the alcoholic epileptics to change jobs more frequently than the other groups. In other words epileptic alcoholic prisoners are different from other alcoholic prisoners in that they turn to crime earlier, make more suicidal attempts and perhaps have even less job stability. It is difficult to suggest why this might be so but it seems possible that if an epileptic man takes to drink in an

Table 36   Analysis of Variance

	Epileptics				Controls				F	P
	Alcoholics		Others		Alcoholics		Others			
	Mean	s.d.	Mean	s.d.	Mean	s.d.	Mean	s.d.		
Age (yr)	29·4	11·1	28·5	10·2	28·6	10·2	27·0	9·3	0·9	NS
Degree of violence	0·8	1·8	0·5	1·3	1·1	2·1	0·9	2·0	1·8	NS
No. of jobs*	2·9	1·5	2·7	1·6	2·4	2·0	2·3	1·5	2·3	(0·1)
Degree unemployment*	1·5	1·1	1·6	1·8	1·4	1·6	1·3	1·6	0·7	NS
No. of pre cons	6·6	5·3	5·9	4·6	7·1	4·1	6·6	5·4	0·8	NS
Age at 1st offence	17·0	8·6	17·1	8·1	27·1	25·0	19·3	17·6	6·6	0·001
No. of violent cons	0·7	1·3	0·4	0·9	0·5	0·9	0·4	0·8	1·8	NS
No. of suic. attempts	1·2	2·0	0·8	1·5	0·8	1·7	0·3	1·0	4·9	0·005

*See p. 82.

attempt to blot out his problems then the effects of the problems already created by the epilepsy and the problems created by the drinking are additive in their destructiveness.

Neurological Examination

In addition to the mental state examination and the questions about drinking habits each man was submitted to a brief neurological check. The following features were observed for each prisoner:
gait (abnormalities from joint or bone disease were excluded)
tendon jerks
power in limbs
speech defects
skull
eye movements
It was at first hoped that each of these items could be analysed separately but it soon became apparent that abnormalities occurred too infrequently for this to be done and so the samples were simply divided into two broad categories (a) those without neurological abnormalities and (b) those with abnormalities.

The findings from the psychiatric data, i.e. the finding that the epileptic group contained 4 brain damaged men and the control group none, led to the prediction that a greater number of probands than controls will have one or more neurological abnormalities. This is confirmed (Table 37) and it can be readily seen that even if the 4 cases of obvious head injury are removed there are still over 3 times as many patients with abnormalities among the epileptics as among the non-epileptics. Such broad figures are relatively meaningless unless we specify what type of abnormalities were detected and this is done in Table 38. An examination of this table shows that a wide range of abnormalities was detected. It also indicates that the epileptic group

Table 37 Neurological Abnormalities

	No neurological abnormalities	Neurological abnormalities	Total
Epileptics	99 (62·7%)	59 (37·3%)	158 (100%)
Controls	160 (89·4%)	19 (10·6%)	179 (100%)

$$X^2 = 33·70 \text{ (1 d.f.) } p<0·0005$$
(Data were missing for 1 control)

Table 38   Types of Neurological Abnormalities Found

Neurological Abnormality	Epileptics		Controls N = 178	
	No.	% of total	No.	% of total
Nystagmus (involuntary eye movements)	34	(21·5)	8	(4·5)
Slurred speech	10	(6·3)	5	(2·8)
Weakness or spasticity of one side of body	9	(5·7)	5	(2·8)
Generalised depression of reflexes	9	(5·7)	4	(2·2)
Skull deformity or defect	6	(3·8)	1	(0·6)
Generalised increases in reflexes	5	(3·2)	1	(0·6)
Depressed reflexes one side	4	(2·5)	3	(1·7)
Increased reflexes one side	4	(2·5)	1	(0·6)
Weakness of external eye muscles	3	(1·9)	3	(1·7)
Blindness in one eye	2	(1·3)	1	(0·6)
Severe stammer	2	(1·3)	1	(0·6)
Personality changes following frontal lobe damage	2	(1·3)	0	
Dragging of both feet	1	(0·6)	0	
Drooping eyelid — one side	1	(0·6)	0	
Facial palsy	1	(0·6)	0	
Severed nerves in arm	0		1	(0·6)

suffered a considerable number of defects which could be attributed to their medication (nystagmus and slurred speech for example), or their high state of anxiety which has already been noted. Clearly such abnormalities constitute a degree of handicap for the individuals concerned but for the purposes of this analysis it is necessary, as before, to take possible drug effects into account. None of the control prisoners was taking a medicine which could have induced these features. Therefore we can remove from the epileptic group all those cases in which it is possible to argue that the neurological abnormalities are secondary to anticonvulsants or an abnormal mental state. Thirty-five cases fall into this category leaving us with 24 other epileptic cases showing neurological abnormality. If now we substitute the 24 cases for the 59 in Table 37, we can retest the proportional difference for significance and find that it is still less than the 5% level of probability ($X^2 = 4·73$ 1 d.f.) and so even allowing for drug induced effects it can still be concluded that the epileptics have more neurological abnormalities than their non-epileptic counterparts.

   To find one tenth of the controls suffering from neurological abnormalities is surprising but it must be re-emphasised that the control sample was not necessarily random for the whole prison population, there may be special reasons for these particular men residing in prisons attended by full-time doctors, reasons which would tend to increase the number of all kinds of abnormalities. Consequently any significant differences found between the groups are especially significant, but the absolute value of features found amongst the controls cannot be taken as representative of all non-epileptic prisoners.

Relationships to Offence Patterns

There were no relationships between the degree of violence in the present offence, the number of previous convictions, or the age at first offence and possessing a neurological abnormality in either group.

Relationship to Type of Epilepsy

A cross tabulation has been made between the epileptic diagnostic categories and neurological abnormalities (Table 39). This reveals that the "other focal" group is strongly associated with neurological abnormality, the "temporal" group less strongly and the "subcortical" groups hardly at all. This is entirely consistent with clinical expectations.

Table 39   Neurological Abnormalities in the Epileptic Subcategories

	Abnormality		
	No	Yes	Totals
Subcortical	19 (82·6%)	4 (17·4%)	23 (100%)
Temporal	28 (58·3%)	20 (41·7%)	48 (100%)
Other focal	12 (38·7%)	19 (61·3%)	31 (100%)
Unrateable	40 (71·4%)	16 (28·6%)	56 (100%)

$$X^2 = 13·74 \ (3 \ \text{d.f.}) \ p < 0.005$$

Discussion

These data indicate a higher level of both psychiatric and neurological abnormality among the epileptic prisoners than among the control prisoners. However, the idea that the psychiatric symptomatology would be especially pronounced in the temporal lobe group is not borne out for the group studied here. Taken in conjunction with the earlier findings (p. 53) that the temporal lobe epileptics are not especially violent in their current offence and are no more likely to have committed a violent offence in the past, this survey gives an interesting contrast to the often quoted view that it is the temporal lobe epileptic who is especially prone to psychiatric disorder and violent behaviour.

It is not the only study to fail to demonstrate this relationship. Guerrant et al. (1968) compared psychomotor epileptics with idiopathic epileptics and with patients suffering from chronic medical diseases. They both found epileptic groups to have a high level of psychiatric disorder although the idiopathic group had a specially high prevalence of personality disorder notably aggressiveness, suspiciousness and negativism. Small and her colleagues (Small et al., 1962; Small et al., 1966; Stevens, 1966) found the same prevalence of sociopathic personality in temporal lobe and non-temporal lobe epileptics and also that different diagnostic subtypes of epilepsy were admitted to hospital at much the same rates. More recently Mignonne et al. (1970) compared temporal lobe and other epileptics attending the National Institute of Neurological Diseases and Strokes in the U.S.A. They found very few distinguishing features in the temporal lobe cases, in particular temporal lobe epilepsy did not seem to be related to schizophrenia, aggressive impulsivity, sexual dysfunction or affective disorder.

How do we explain these discrepancies? Firstly, it should be emphasised that almost every epileptic population which is studied has been through some sort of selection procedure (the sample considered here is no exception). It may be, for example, that antisocial temporal lobe epileptics with affective or suicidal symptoms are less likely to go to prison than other sorts of psychiatrically disturbed antisocial epileptics, thereby pushing up the level of antisocial temporal lobe epilepsy cases in other samples. Secondly, psychiatric 'disability' is frequently used as a generic term for a conglomerate of symptoms which may not necessarily be inter-correlated e.g. aggressiveness, intellectual dysfunction, depression. The findings of this study relate to affective symptoms (which in itself is an addition of depressive and anxiety symptoms), suicidal feelings and suicide attempts. Perhaps this point can be illustrated by reference to the study of Oxford head injury material made by Lishman (1968). He found that in his material there was a clear relationship between severity of psychiatric disability (a composite of intellectual, behavioural and emotional disturbances) and temporal lobe damage. If only the severely psychiatrically disturbed cases were considered (21% of his material) then affective disorders, behavioural disorders and somatic complaints (when taken as individual categories) were all more frequent *after frontal* lobe damage than after damage elsewhere. However, temporal lobe damage was still especially associated with intellectual disturbance. The Oxford study also gives us a clue to a third possible explanation. The level at which the investigator sets his cut off point may influence the findings for relationships between foci of cerebral disturbance and psychiatric disability. It may be that as far as behaviour disturbance is concerned imprisonment indicates a high level of disorder and therefore cannot, perhaps, be reasonably compared with hospital samples. It is even possible that the epileptics studied here have suffered either before or during imprisonment such severe stress and disturbance that subtle reactions to having one sort of epilepsy as opposed to another have been overwhelmed and become less significant. Even so, it is worth noting that this study did find a positive relationship between temporal lobe epilepsy and reported suicidal behaviour in the past.

Recently a comprehensive review on the association between temporal lobe epilepsy and aggression has appeared (Kligman and Goldberg, 1975). They point to the immense difficulties in finding operational definitions for both temporal lobe epilepsy and for aggression and in their analysis of the studies published to date indicate that sample bias and lack of regard for the reliability and validity of behavioural assessments devalue the findings reported in many cases.

There is no justification to generalise from the current study to others, nor to comment about global concepts of "psychiatric disability" and epilepsy. It simply appears that epileptics in prison have a high level of affective symptomatology, higher indeed than the already high level suffered by other prisoners. It emerges that this cannot be attributed to their medication, nor is it an especial feature of any one sort of epileptic prisoner. Epileptics in prison carry, moreover, an especial suicidal risk, which may be related to temporal lobe epilepsy.

It is impossible to deduce from these data the reason for the increased proportion of affective symptoms, we might guess that social rejection, distorted self image and brain dysfunction all play their part. There may even be special prison stresses for the epileptic. Certainly many of the men in the current survey saw themselves as underprivileged even by prison standards. They do, for example, have special protective restrictions applied to them and they are unlikely to get to the specialised training prisons. They can often be the object of derision (nicknamed 'fitters' and 'eppies') in the harsh subculture that exists among prison inmates.

Turning to drinking behaviour we find that in this survey 15-17% of both epileptic and non-epileptic prisoners were rated as alcoholic with just over 40% being regarded as excessively heavy drinkers. This fits remarkably closely to the overall findings discovered by Gibbens and Silberman (1970) in their prison survey. The similarity between the groups in drinking behaviour and alcoholic symptomatology suggests that epileptic prisoners are no more or less prone to suffer from alcohol abuse than are other prisoners. Perhaps it should be noted in passing that over a quarter of the population survey here have shown at least one symptom of addictive alcoholism in their lives: by any token a point of considerable medical interest.

An analysis of variance indicates that there is very little relationship between alcoholism and the other factors examined in the survey which distinguished the epileptics from the non-epileptics. It appears that the control non-epileptics are less likely to have made a suicide attempt than any of the other groups, but in other respects they are remarkably similar to the other prisoners. The alcoholic control prisoners stand out from the other groups in terms of the late onset of their official criminality. This is no great surprise when it is realised that alcoholism itself is a disorder with an insidious onset and severe secondary problems often appear only after it has been established for some time. The progression of rates of suicide attempts from non-alcoholic controls to epileptic alcoholics is striking. It would appear that as further pathology is added, either epilepsy or alcoholism, the attempted suicide rate goes up.

CHAPTER 6

Social Factors

In previous chapters straight comparisons have been made between
the epileptic prisoners and the non-epileptic prisoners. If we are now
to examine social or environmental factors we have two major
problems. Firstly environmental factors are difficult to measure with
accuracy and it could be argued that in a retrospective study this
should not even be attempted. However it seems reasonable to assume
that provided very simple questions which have some chance of a valid
answer are posed, and provided results are examined with sufficient
circumspection the advantages (mainly in terms of generating
hypotheses) outweigh the dangers. Secondly a straight comparison
between two kinds of prisoners is unlikely to be very fruitful for social
issues because the fact of imprisonment is likely to produce close
matching on environmental parameters. In an attempt to meet this
second point to some extent a second control group was investigated
after the main prison survey was over. By courtesy of two consultant
colleagues access was obtained to the epilepsy clinic at the Maudsley
Hospital and the neurological Clinic at Kings College Hospital.

Hospital Sample

Using the method described earlier a consecutive sample of male
epileptics between the ages of 16 and 65 years was interviewed.
Patients were excluded who suffered from dementia or who had been
in trouble with the law other than for one or two non-indictable
motoring offences. All the cases referred were designated "definitely

epileptic" by their consultants, were fully investigated and fitted the diagnostic criteria given earlier. By this process 67 cases were selected and they therefore formed a second control group of non-criminal epileptics.

It has earlier been emphasised that sampling frames of this kind cannot produce a representative sample of epileptics, they have already been pre-selected by hospital referral processes. In this particular case the sample is biased towards including patients with psychological problems and abnormal mental states, since the Maudsley is a mental hospital. This bias is a slight advantage, as it means that members of this control group, like the probands, have more than one handicap — epilepsy plus antisocial behaviour for the probands, epilepsy plus psychological disturbance for the non-prisoners.

As previously demonstrated the two prison samples were well matched for age and criminal history. Unfortunately, however, the hospital sample could not be so carefully controlled. When the prisoner and hospital epileptics were compared on a number of simple clinical features a significant difference emerged (Table 40) in respect

Table 40   (N.B. Two or three cases have been omitted from each sub-total because of missing data)

	Epileptic prisoners (N = 158)	Hospital epileptics	X^2	Non-epileptic prisoners (N = 180)
Heavy drinkers	73 (46%)	7 (10%)	24·17	74 (41%)
No psychiatric abnormality	68 (43%)	32 (48%)	NS	106 (59%)
Severe psychiatric abnormality	51 (31%)	14 (21%)	NS	28 (16%)
Neurological abnormality	58 (37%)	30 (45%)	NS	19 (11%)
Suicidal ideas	18 (11%)	5 (8%)	NS	6 (3%)

of drinking behaviour. Furthermore the similarity between the groups in terms of psychiatric symptoms disguised a number of qualitative differences. There were no psychotic prisoners but two such hospital cases, there were no prisoners with a degree of dementia but three such hospital cases, 21 per cent of the prisoner epileptics expressed anxiety symptoms but only 9 per cent of the hospital cases did so.

Table 41 indicates the assessment of epileptic type in the two groups. Table 42 illustrates the most serious difference between the groups, the hospital patients being significantly older than the prisoner epileptics. To allow for or partial out any effect of age, the subsequent results have been set out in age groups and Cochran's test (Maxwell), which determines a critical ratio (CR), applied to each pair of comparisons.

Table 41   Types of Epilepsy

	Epileptic prisoners	Hospital epileptics
Subcortical	23 (23%)	9 (16%)
Temporal	48 (47%)	28 (51%)
Other focal	31 (30%)	18 (33%)
N.K.	56	12

$$X^2 = 0.46 \ (2 \text{ d.f.}) \text{ NS}$$

All 3 groups were examined in terms of 6 social measures (i) social class, (ii) material conditions in the childhood home, (iii) sibship size, (iv) parental loss, (v) occupational record, (vi) marital status.

Social class: The system used was the somewhat unsatisfactory but commonly recognised Registrar-General's scale of occupations (General Register Office, 1960). I. Professional and like; II. Occupations intermediate between I and III; III. Skilled occupations; IV. Partly skilled occupations; V. Unskilled occupations.

Table 42   Age Structure of the three samples

	Non-Epileptic prisoners	Epileptic prisoners	Hospital epileptics
16-25 years	94*	76	26
26-35 ,,	47	45	13
36-45 ,,	29	20	12
46 + ,,	10	17	16
Total	180	158	67
Mean	27·7	28·9	34·6
S.D.	9·77	10·62	14·15

*One 15-year old non-epileptic prisoner has been omitted from subsequent calculations.

The pros and cons of using this particular classification have been examined by Glass (1954). In using such a scale, however, it is important to specify which member of a family is to determine the classification and at which point in time. For example, does the son of a doctor, who at one time held down a job as a supermarket manager, but recently has only been able to obtain employment as a barman, fall into Class I, II or IV? Such problems cannot entirely be circumvented, but the following scheme has been adopted throughout. The occupation of the prisoner's *de facto* father was noted; here the *de facto* father was defined as the person who supported or tried to support the prisoner for the largest part of his childhood (before the age of 16), and could therefore be either his real father, his stepfather, the man his mother was living with, or even his mother, according to circumstances. His job was taken as the one which he was reported to have held for the longest period in his working life. Prisoners brought up in institutions without a year or more of family life were counted as 'others', along with servicemen's children.

Table 43 indicates that the 3 groups come from differing social background. Almost half of the non-epileptic prisoners came from homes where father was a semi-skilled or unskilled worker, and this was the case for approximately one third of the epileptic prisoners, but for only one fifth of the hospital epileptics. The prisoner epileptics fell mid-way between the other two groups and the differences between them and the other groups are significant.

Table 43   Fathers work by social class

Age	Non-epileptic prisoners		Epileptic prisoners		Hospital epileptics	
	I, II, III	IV, V	I, II, III	IV, V	I, II, III	IV, V
16-25	46	40	39	26	21	4
26-35	21	22	26	12	11	2
36-45	16	12	13	4	9	3
46 +	6	3	7	8	10	5
Total	89 (54%)	77 (46%)	85 (63%)	50 (37%)	51 (79%)	14 (22%)

13 non-epileptic prisoners, 23 epileptic prisoners, and 2 hospital epileptics have been omitted because of missing data.

CR between epileptic prisoners and non-epileptic prisoners = 2·42 ($p < 0.05$)
CR between epileptic prisoners and hospital epileptics   = 2·42 ($p < 0.05$)

Childhood home: Each man was asked if the home in which he spent the longest part of his childhood (0-16 years) included a bathroom to which the family had access, or if at any stage he had to share a bed with another member of the household for a month or longer. Any man who had spent 15 or more years of his childhood in an institution was put into a separate category and excluded from the analysis. This accommodation rating did not distinguish between the groups.

Sibship size: Each man was also asked the size of his sibship, including himself, half siblings, foster siblings and adoptive siblings who lived in the household for twelve months or more during his childhood.

Both groups of prisoners were more likely to have come from big families than the hospital epileptics (Table 44).

Table 44   Total number of siblings reared together in childhood home

Age	Non-epileptic prisoners		Epileptic prisoners		Hospital epileptics	
	0-4	5 +	0-4	5 +	0-4	5 +
16-25	53	39	52	23	25	1
26-35	31	16	20	22	12	1
36-45	15	14	7	12	10	12
46 +	6	3	11	6	10	6
Total	105 (59%)	72 (41%)	90 (59%)	63 (41%)	57 (85%)	10 (15%)

2 non-epileptic prisoners, 5 epileptic prisoners have been omitted, because of missing data

CR between epileptic prisoners and non-epileptic prisoners = 0·24 (NS)
CR between epileptic prisoners and hospital epileptics   = 4·14 ($p < 0·01$)

Parental loss: Parental loss was defined as the continuous absence of one or both natural parents for at least 12 consecutive months before the child's 15th birthday, excluding periods of absence entirely related to residence in a penal institution (e.g. an approved school), as these are imposed from outside the family and cannot be considered as aetiological factors.

This broad definition was chosen not because of any preconceptions about the significance of separation as such, but simply as a reasonably objective measure of significant family disruption in childhood, fully accepting that it includes a heterogenous collection of psychological and physical insults, from deprivation of example to rejection, poverty, and institutionalisations. (See also Greer *et al.*, 1966). The age at which paternal loss was said to have begun was also noted.

Unfortunately the study of childhood and early family life by retrospective inquiry is fraught with hazards. One is usually relying upon both co-operation and accuracy of memory. A study very relevant here was carried out in 1964 by Yarrow *et al.* They were fortunate in having some contemporary baseline data on mother-child relationships and child characteristics from a nursery school and they were able to re-interview 226 of the mothers of these children, some 28 years later, to compare their recall of the childhood events with the recordings made at the time. They found significant correspondence between the baseline data and the mothers' reports, but the relationships were disappointingly low in magnitude, the median correlation co-efficient between initial and recall data being only 0·37. The more factual observations were recalled with greater reliability than the judgemental ones. Clearly, however, conclusions drawn from such retrospective data must be very tentative and must never be taken in isolation. Reassuringly, recall of parental separation was the most reliable measure of childhood experience Yarrow *et al.* could find ($r = 0·72$ for fathers and $r = 0·44$ for mothers).

High levels of parental loss before the sixteenth birthday were encountered in all three groups, but there is a gradation between the hospital epileptics (40% of whom had suffered such a difficulty), the epileptic prisoners (56%) and the non-epileptic prisoners (65%). The differences between the prisoner epileptics and the other groups do not quite reach the 5% level of significance (Table 45). The age at which

Table 45   Parental Loss before 16th birthday

Age	Non-Ep Prisoners		Epileptic Prisoners		Hospital Epileptics	
	No loss	Loss	No Loss	Loss	No Loss	Loss
16-25	27	64	35	39	16	10
26-35	13	31	12	32	7	6
36 +	21	16	20	14	17	11
Total	61 (35%)	111 (65%)	67 (44%)	85 (56%)	40 (60%)	27 (40%)

(6 epileptic prisoners and 7 non-epileptic prisoners have been omitted because of missing data.)

CR between ep prisoners and non-ep prisoners   =   1·65 ($p<0·1$)
CR between ep prisoners and hospital epileptics   =   1·75 ($p<0·1$)

the mother loss and the age at which the father loss occurred was similar for all three groups, 40-50% of the men having lost their mothers before their fifth birthday and 55-65% having lost their father at this time.

Occupational record: Two scales were used. Each man was asked for as full an account as possible of his occupational history for the five years preceding his reception into prison. Young men with less than five years potential history were rated on the total of their working life, unless this was less than 12 months in which event their case was discarded. Severe recidivists who had worked for less than five years in the preceding 10 because of imprisonment were rate on the full 10 years.

The two scales were:

(a) the average number of different jobs per year, using three points, 1 or less, 2 or 3, 4 or more; a change of job being rated whenever a man moved from one *employer* to another;

(b) the percentage of time spent unemployed (other than in prison or hospital) using a four-point scale, 0-5%, 26-50%, 51% or more.

Looking at the work history of the interviewees themselves there is a trend for the epileptic prisoners to change jobs more frequently than the other prisoners, but there is a sharp distinction between both sorts of prisoners and the hospital epileptics, who are much more stable in terms of job movements (Table 46). Interestingly, however, the proportion of time spent unemployed does not distinguish between the groups.

Table 46   Average number of jobs per year

Age	Non-epileptic prisoners		Epileptic prisoners		Hospital epileptics	
	1 or 2/yr	3 + /yr	1 or 2/yr	3 + /yr	1 or 2/yr	3 + /yr
16-25	43	44	27	45	19	0
26-35	25	19	20	20	11	1.
36-45	13	14	6	13	12	0
46 +	4	3	7	7	10	2
Total	85 (52%)	80 (49%)	60 (41%)	85 (59%)	52 (95%)	3 (5%)

14 non-epileptic prisoners, 13 epileptic prisoners and 12 hospital epileptics have been omitted because of missing data.

CR between epileptic prisoners and non-epileptic prisoners = 1·92 ($p<0·1$)

The hospital epileptics are obviously different from other groups.

Marital status: A distinction was made between single men and the remainder. A man was counted as *de facto* married if he had had any heterosexual co-habitation lasting for six consecutive months or longer.

Although all three groups had a high proportion of unmarried individuals, there were no differences between them (range 57-61%).

Discussion

In terms of the social characteristics, the similarities between all three groups are more striking than the differences. It is interesting, for example, that there were no significant differences between the groups in respect of unemployment suffered in recent years, the high level of single men, or the physical conditions of the childhood home. This last finding is perhaps a little surprising in view of the differences that were found between the groups for father's social class.

From the childhood factors it would appear that the non-epileptic prisoners come from less well off background than either of the other two groups, almost half of them having fathers working in social groups IV or V although the material circumstances of childhood measured in housing terms did not distinguish between the groups (perhaps such measures are too crude). The sibship size (which will be seen by some as an indicator of the parental resources, both economic and emotional, available to each child) indicated that both groups of prisoners come from larger families than the hospital group.

In summary there is a social class gradation from the non-epileptic prisoners, to the epileptic prisoners, to the hospital epileptics. There is also a gradation in family size from the hospital epileptics to both groups of prisoners. Parental loss experiences showed a similar trend with the prisoner non-epileptics faring worst, followed by the epileptic prisoners, and once again the hospital epileptics coming out best. In occupational terms however there was a trend for the epileptic prisoners to have less job stability than the other groups. Overall it appears that where differences occur it tends to be in terms of the hospital epileptics having better social environments (in childhood) than the prisoner groups. This is no great surprise as we know that childhood social factors are important determinants of later delinquency (e.g. West and Farrington, 1973). This point will be discussed later but here it is worth noting that the epileptic prisoners were not differentiated sharply from their prisoner controls in terms of social background. Where there are differences they are mostly in terms of the epileptic prisoners suffering slightly fewer disadvantages than the non-epileptic prisoners. If imprisonment is, at least in part, a symptom of social malfunction then this finding is not very surprising for it suggests that social disadvantages and medical disadvantages are additive in producing that malfunction.

CHAPTER 7

Discussion

The first objective of this inquiry was to determine the prevalence of epilepsy in English prisons. This seems to be between 7 and 8 per 1000 men which is higher than any of the recent estimates for the condition in the general population. Examination of the more detailed part of the survey suggests that this is by no means an over-estimate of the number in custody and may even be an under-estimate. It is the younger epileptic men and those over 45 years who show particular liability to imprisonment. Over half the men in the survey had never attended an epileptic clinic, over a quarter had never had an EEG, and one fifth were receiving no anti-convulsant treatment at the time of their reception into prison.

The second objective of the inquiry has been to examine some of the ways in which a representative group of epileptic prisoners differ from other prisoners in the hope that this will illuminate some of their special problems, both past and present, and perhaps even generate hypotheses about the relationship, if any, between epilepsy and imprisonment.

The close matching achieved by taking the next prisoner in the admission register to each epileptic has meant that the probands and the controls were also matched for type of offence and therefore little could be said in confirmation or refutation of the oft quoted hypothesis that epileptics are more likely to commit violent offences than other criminals.

Interviewing men in prison and validating the information obtained presents immense problems but the simple techniques used here give rise to the optimistic view that these difficulties can be at least partially surmounted, and that meaningful surveys of this type are credible.

An operational definition of epilepsy, arbitrarily chosen has shown good reliability when applied to these data, and about one third of the cases examined were classified, with some confidence, as of the temporal lobe type of epilepsy. Unfortunately not enough is known about the expected proportion of temporal lobe cases in the general population to tell whether this is a particularly important finding. A point of considerable clinical interest however was the remarkably low number of cases, designated as epileptic by the Prison Medical Department, without grand mal seizures. This was taken as confirmation of their own verbal assurances that they tend to under-diagnose the condition rather than over-diagnose in cases of doubt, and as evidence for regarding the prevalence found in the initial census as a minimal estimate.

An important aspect of an epileptic prisoner population is its level of alcoholism because it is generally thought that epilepsy and alcoholism are related, and likewise alcoholism and criminality are related. In this survey 15-17% of both groups were rated as alcoholic, and when individual symptoms were studied there was again remarkable similarity. Therefore no adjustments were thought necessary to exclude a significant number of men from the proband group who were primarily alcoholic and only secondarily epileptic. In addition to alcoholism a few general psychiatric features were looked at because there is evidence that suggests that epileptics are particularly prone to suffer with affective disturbances and to make suicidal attempts. These points were confirmed for this group, as was the notion that it is the temporal lobe epileptic who is particularly prone to suffer anxiety and depression.

Crime and Epilepsy

The whole process of stereotyping and stigmatising particular groups in society as especially likely to commit crimes is not only morally repugnant; it is scientific nonsense. On the other hand there is the finding in this survey of an excess prevalence of epilepsy in prison. Part of the confusion clears when it is realised that prisons are institutions and a very important part of the whole complex of institutional care in this country which embraces mental hospitals, common lodging houses, colonies, hostels and the like (Gunn, 1974). As long ago as

1939 Penrose was collecting evidence suggesting that prison and mental hospital populations are interrelated in some way. It is possible therefore that we are simply observing in this survey that epileptics are a bit more prone to need institutional care than healthy members of the population. The Victorians acknowledged as much by building epileptic colonies.

Asylums traditionally have looked after numbers of epileptics and will no doubt continue to do so if they are allowed to remain in existence. However Bowden (1975) has shown recently that because of policy changes and financial stringencies within the National Health Service increasing numbers of patients are being diverted from mental hospitals to security institutions, especially prisons, especially if they show any behavioural difficulties.

It cannot be emphasised too strongly that this survey cannot give definite answers to any questions about a possible association between epilepsy and crime. All that can be said from these data is that there is an excess number of epileptics residing in British prisons. This could be for one of two fundamental reasons (even allowing for the institutional cross-over mentioned above). Firstly it may be that epileptics commit more crimes which can be punished by imprisonment than other citizens. Secondly, it may be that epileptics, whilst having similar crime rates to the general population are more likely to be sentenced to imprisonment. Neither of these hypotheses can be tested by a prison survey, a court survey would be required. However, given that one or both of these factors must be operating it is possible to speculate about underlying mechanisms.

Firstly it is clear from this survey that epileptics are not getting to prison specially frequently because of automatic behaviour. Whilst there is evidence that, rarely, automatic crimes can occur, they did not account for one single conviction in this series of prisoners. One basic fear that the epileptic is liable to lapse into an uncontrollable fugue-like state in which he will undertake antisocial perhaps dangerous acts has been greatly exaggerated.

There seem to be at present 5 possible ways in which imprisonment and epilepsy can be associated other than by chance.

A.   Courts have a bias toward institutionalising epileptics when they have committed offences, and increasingly this is meaning imprisonment.

B.   Brain function can, in certain individuals be responsible for both the epilepsy and the antisocial behaviour.

C.   Epilepsy generates special social and psychological problems (e.g.

rejection, feelings of inferiority) which in their turn lead to anti-social reactions.

D.   Harmful social factors such as parental neglect and the like lead to an excess prevalence of both epilepsy and antisocial behaviour simultaneously.

E.   Harmful social factors lead to behaviour disturbances which produce not only conflict with the law but also accidents and self neglect which in turn sometimes lead on to cerebral damage and epilepsy.

Each of these hypotheses will be discussed in turn with illustrations, where possible, from the case material of the survey.

A. *Differential Imprisonment*

It is precisely in the area of court practice where it is impossible to draw conclusions without a court survey. All that can be noted here is that some of the epileptic prisoners believed that their epilepsy contributed towards getting a prison sentence. Some claimed that other people convicted with them only received fines or probation. Obviously such comments could not be checked and the sentences may have been differentiated on other grounds. This hypothesis will therefore have to be left without further comment, although it may be worth noting that for some of the cases quoted in subsequent sections it can be argued that a medical disposal would have been as appropriate as imprisonment.

B. *Brain Malfunction*

Grunberg and Pond (1957) compared 53 selected epileptic children who had conduct disorders with 53 psychologically normal epileptic children, and 35 conduct disordered non-epileptic children attending the Maudsley Hospital. They defined conduct disorders in terms of severe and frequent temper tantrums, destructiveness, fighting, truanting, wandering, lying, stealing, etc. and were able to show that the 2 epileptic groups differed in the proportions of disturbing environmental factors they had suffered, whilst the disturbed epileptics did not differ significantly from the disturbed non-epileptics in these respects. Surprisingly however they were unable to distinguish between the epileptics and the non-epileptics on their measures of underlying brain damage (perinatal cerebral damage, meningitis, encephalitis). The authors comment on this puzzling finding and point out that it could well be due to a selection bias. It would be illogical to conclude that epilepsy and behaviour disorder are never related via cerebral factors for that is equivalent to saying that cerebral malfunction and behaviour are never related.

In a more recent study Bagley (1971) set out to replicate the Grunberg and Pond work using a group of children attending a neurological clinic. He compared 83 disturbed epileptic children with 83 disturbed non-epileptics, from a child guidance clinic matching them for sex, social class, age, aggressiveness and anxiety. He also compared 35 normal epileptic children with 35 matched normal non-epileptics. Bagley constructed two measures of brain injury (i) birth difficulties and (ii) blind EEG interpretations. Using either of these as an indicator of cerebral damage he was able to distinguish between normal and aggressive children. Interestingly he found no relationship between temporal lobe damage and aggression; this is different from the viewpoint, and the studies quoted earlier but is in keeping with the present study.

In the current study just over a third of the epileptic group exhibited central nervous system signs which were picked out by a brief and superficial neurological examination but no correlation could be obtained between this measure and either degree of violence, or degree of impulsivity. A significant but weak relationship was demonstrated between neurological signs and the degree of unemployment suffered.

The five severely brain damaged individuals have already been mentioned in Chapter 5. "Edward" illustrates the kind of case in which the antisocial behaviour can probably best be viewed as almost entirely caused by cerebral damage. A 39 year-old man with an apparently normal childhood in a well integrated working class home, he suffered no rejection, "parental loss" or other significant trauma until the age of 29 years. There was no previous history of head injury but at the age of 29 years he was involved in a motor-cycle accident sustaining a long linear partially depressed fracture of his skull together with a fracture of the roof of the orbit of his right eye. Some ten days later he still had cerebro-spinal fluid coming down his nose and he had developed meningitis. With the aid of neurosurgery he gradually recovered, his right-sided weakness and his disorientation receding slowly. After leaving hospital he attempted to return to his wife and to his old job as a welder but he failed completely, soon degenerating into an unemployed drifter, stealing frequently and sleeping either in the street or in hostels for casuals. Since his accident there have been fifteen indictable offences recorded (all for stealing) in ten years, and he has received a total of seven years ten months imprisonment besides other punishments. His mental state at examination showed excessive jocularity, over-familiarity, easy provocation to tears or laughter, mildly paranoid ideas about "niggers" and garrulousness. His fits began with an aura of nausea and rapidly went into a *grand mal* seizure during which he was incontinent. In prison his fits were well controlled (perhaps two or three attacks per year) with the aid of phenobarbitone/phenytoin mixture. He claimed to take this outside prison as well, but this is extremely unlikely in view of his disorderd existence and of the fact that he had no regular doctor.

It is emphasised that this man's behaviour can be *almost* entirely accounted for by his brain damage, but not quite, for a closer examination of his record shows that as a boy of fourteen he was brought before the magistrate for "borrowing" a bike which didn't belong to him, his sister also stole something once, and at the time of the road accident he was driving the motor cycle, and to a minor extent we can see an element of the "consequential" case history (see below).

Another example of clear cut cerebral damage syndrome also gives a hint of an interaction effect. "Frank" was brought up in unfortunate circumstances by an alcoholic father and a sick mother who died when he was nine years old, managed to settle down in his twenties by joining the army where he learnt a trade, gained promotion and found a fiancee. He had had no head injuries or epilepsy in childhood but had run away from home several times and had sustained one conviction for stealing when thirteen years old. At the age of 25 he was in the back of an army lorry which crashed, received severe injuries to the top of his skull, and was admitted to hospital deeply comatose. After a week he regained consciousness and over the next few weeks a partial blindness gradually cleared, up, although he needed many weeks treatment with pitressin tannate for an inability to concentrate his urine, caused by damage to the pituitary gland in his skull. Following the accident he suffered recurrent *grand mal* epileptic seizures heralded by a feeling of "blankness" in his head. These were reasonably controlled in prison by phenobarbitone/phenytoin mixture, but outside he was an unemployed vagrant. Attempts to help him in a mental hospital and an epileptic colony have failed because he persistently absconded. Since his accident 22 offences have been recorded; two for drunkenness, three for loitering and being on enclosed premises; the remainder for stealing offences of various sorts.

Again the antisocial behaviour is probably best seen as a function of his severe cerebral damage but here, in keeping with the viewpoint of Jarvie (1954 and 1958), we are probably seeing potential behaviour released into actuality by the loss of some sort of inhibiting mechanism.

C. *Psycho-Social Problems*

The survey has clearly demonstrated that as a group the epileptic prisoners admitted more anxiety and depressive symptoms at interview than the non-epileptic and had in the past more frequently attempted suicide. These features cannot immediately be attributed to the unfortunate pressures which society imposes upon epileptics although it would be logical to see some of the symptoms in that light, especially as one or two of the patients interviewed attributed their worries and misery to their epilepsy.

e.g. *"George"* "No one will give you a chance"
"I only have little fits"
"Still I suppose I might hit someone one day"
"Do you think I've got cancer, doctor?"

"Harry" "We eps don't get a square deal—we are looked upon as scum"
"My greatest ambition is to get rid of these fits so that I can get a job like other people".

"Ivan" "I'm looked upon as the black sheep of the family. The trouble is I can't get a proper job—they won't have me at home anymore, they even refuse to send their address to the prison governor".

Admittedly such comments could be a function of the mental state at interview rather than related to reality but most clinicians will have met some patients with this kind of problem. In the last example "Ivan's" statement was quite correct.

Graham and Rutter whose survey of children on the Isle of Wight has been mentioned before concluded when studying the epileptic children that:

"The widespread community prejudice against epilepsy was probably an adverse factor in the epileptic child's development and it may have been one reason for the high rate of (psychiatric) disorder in the epileptic group."

They point out that supportive evidence for his notion comes from the slightly higher rate of psychiatric disorder (50%) of those whose physical activities had been restricted, compared with the rate in the remainder (33%).

"John" was a young borstal lad who had epilepsy since the age of three years. His home was a stable well-integrated one. There was no family history of epilepsy or behaviour disorder and the origins of his attacks were unknown although they always appeared to have been focal. *Grand mal* seizures rarely afflicted him (about every 12-18 months) but minor focal attacks (twitching of the left side of his face accompanied by numbness of his left arm) were very frequent indeed, and at the time of the interview he was having five or six every hour, in spite of medication with a mixture of phenobarbitone, phenytoin and primidone. Although his mental state was rated as "normal" it became clear during the session spent with him that he bitterly resented his epilepsy, and felt a failure. Although his IQ was in the bright normal range he was always a shy boy and had never had a very rewarding job (petrol pump boy, builder's labourer, etc). The longest he had ever stayed in one position was four months. He complained that he hadn't a chance of a better job because other people soon noticed that he is "odd" and find out that he is "epileptic". Sometimes he refused to even go and look for a job because he felt humiliated and he was totally opposed to the idea of joining the disabled register at the Labour Exchange. "I'm not disabled", he insisted. To add to his difficulties his parents always found both his behaviour and his condition an enigma, the probation officer reported: "His father is very concerned about his status in the community . . . his attitude vacillates between outright rejection and protective over-indulgence and he finds it difficult to know what to do for the best for his son". The boy himself seemed afraid of his epilepsy, talked at length about his violent feelings and expressed ambivalence towards his home. Several convictions have been recorded from malicious wounding to shopbreaking. Many of the boy's problems are put into clearer perspective when it is realised that his healthy elder brother had made a successful professional career for himself and that the patient was constantly comparing himself with his brother. Here it could be postulated that brain damage is the prime determinant of the behaviour disorder and no doubt it played its part, however it seems more logical to attribute his resentment and his anti-social behaviour to a reaction against a combination of his own self image, his lack of success in comparison to his brother, social prejudice and inconsistent parental handling.

As the survey has clearly shown, severe environmental stress is the rule rather than the exception for this group of men and "Keith" illustrates perhaps a more typical example of an interaction between the epilepsy and the environment in the genesis of anti-social behaviour. This man had had epilepsy of unknown aetiology since infancy. He was brought up in a deprived home having lost his mother during his own childbirth. His invalid father, who had both psychiatric illness and heart trouble, was unable to cope with the family and our subject was brought up by his maternal aunt until father remarried. However the stepmother didn't like the boy and quarrelled with the aunt. Soon the child began to wander from home and his father took him to court as beyond parental contol, which resulted in the boy being sent to a training school. From this time many medical and social work reports are available about him and it is clear from their descriptions that most people who handled him disliked and disbelieved him . . . "From the beginning his poor attitude towards all around him was evident" . . "He could give me no explanation or reason why he was running away from home" . . . "A liar" (statements written by his professional advisors when he was aged eleven). Although he had had seizures for some years, when he was 17 a psychiatrist implied that his illness was a fabrication to get himself into hospital, and to obtain sick benefit (he was admitted to the same hospital in status epilepticus the following year). In her reply to the relatives questionnaire his stepmother said that he had never had fits, seizures or epilepsy. Most of his offences have concerned the theft of small amounts of money. Although he found inter-personal relationships very difficult to handle he managed to maintain a precarious marriage for a few years and at interview his latest offence was a pathetically ineffective attempt to prop this up by agreeing to go back to his wife's home town taking the furniture on HP with them, and stealing the cash from the gas meter to pay for the trip. He received six months imprisonment. Employment was nearly always an impossibility and although he has worked for short periods as a builder's labourer he spent most of his life unemployed. He put the characteristic dilemma neatly into his own words "If you say you're an epileptic, they say, 'Sorry, full up', but if you don't tell them you get sacked at the first fit".

Further elaborations are not necessary to draw several tenable conclusions from this case (a) his background difficulties would have been sufficient to produce antisocial behaviour in many individuals (and indeed his elder brother has become an alcoholic); (b) his epilepsy may well have been caused by the trauma suffered during a difficult childbirth (it was lethal to his mother), (c) he has suffered a good deal of social rejection (much of it "justified" in ordinary terms) which has not assisted his progress. Overall it can be concluded that his epilepsy is clearly not the result of his behaviour, and that cerebral damage is probably only a small contributor to his behaviour disorder.

D. *Environment*

As already noted Grunberg and Pond (1957) found that epileptic children with conduct disorders differed from epileptic children without such disorders in terms of disturbing environmental factors. The epileptics with the behaviour disorders have received more "disturbed maternal attitude", more "disturbed paternal attitude", more "sibling rivalry", more "paternal marital disharmony", more "restriction at home", and more "breaks and changes in their environment" than the psychologically normal epileptics. In contrast however the disturbed epileptics did not differ significantly from the disturbed non-epileptics in these respects. They concluded that "these findings suggest a causal relationship between conduct disorders and disturbed social background in epileptic children." The Bagley study confirmed this finding.

In their Isle of Wight survey Graham and Rutter (1968) demonstrated the validity of this association between environment and behaviour disorder for a wider group of children with organic brain dysfunction (which, of course, included many with epilepsy). They found that adverse familial factors were more frequent among the epileptic children with psychiatric disorder (a combination of neurotic and antisocial disorders). Children with psychiatric disorder were more likely to have mothers who scored more than six items on a specifically devised self-rating questionnaire listing various emotional and psychosomatic complaints. However to have come from a "broken home" (defined as the child living other than with his two natural parents) was not associated with psychiatric disorder.

It can reasonably be expected that families with considerable internal family pathology will be less successful in a whole range of activities than other families. This is to some extent confirmed here by the finding that both prisoner groups had a high level of parental loss (which is postulated as a measure of family pathology) and at the same time came from homes which had been much less successful in the occupational sphere than the hospital sample. Here care must be exercised not to overemphasise this association because it is possible that part of the explanation for the prison population's skew towards the poorer end of the social spectrum is a reflection of legal prejudice e.g. it is conceivable that a boy from an articulate but disturbed home who became involved in a drunken brawl would be dealt with less severely by police and lawyers than a similar boy from a disturbed unskilled home. Nevertheless this is unlikely to be the whole explanattion.

In the past whenever epilepsy has been noted to be associated with disturbances in the environment (Lennox, 1942; WHO, 1957; Bagley, 1969) an hereditary explanation has been postulated. For example, Stein (1933) compared 1000 institutionalised epileptics with 1115 non-epileptics and showed that the family histories of the epileptics contained 2-3 times the proportion of neuropsychiatric disorders as did the controls, Stein concluded that a constitutional weakness was being passed on from ancestor to offspring genetically and that whether or not such a constitutionally weak individual developed seizures depended upon the presence or absence of particular environmental factors, which he didn't elaborate upon. It is noteworthy that when the "total neuropsychiatric" features were broken down into particular categories the relatives disability which distinguished most strongly between the epileptics and the controls was alcoholism in the father. The World Health Organisation's report on juvenile epilepsy decided that "so striking are the associations between severe temporal-lobe behaviour disorders and family background that one is tempted to postulate a genetic or familial factor to account for it. Such an idea is, of course, but a revival of the 'epileptic constitution' but in a new form which may be heuristically more useful". Interestingly, the report does not discuss why the poor family background should apply particularly to temporal lobe epilepsy in which injuries of all types play a very significant role.

Knobloch and Pasamanick (1966) have set out an account of the ways in which biological and socio-cultural factors may interact to prevent an individual achieving his full genotypic potential. They regard pre-natal maternal health as of crucial importance and quote examples from their own work showing that premature infants are more likely to develop "deviations in neurologic patterns". These authors are of course famous for the development of their theory of "reproductive casualty" which they define as "the sequelae of harmful events during pregnancy and parturition resulting in damage to the foetus or new born infant, and primarily localised to the central nervous system" (Knobloch and Pasamanick). When Lilienfield and Pasamanick (1954) examined the pre-natal and para-natal records 374 white epileptic children they found that they showed significantly more complications of pregnancy and delivery, more prematurity and more abnormal neo-natal conditions that a similar number of controls matched for place of birth, race and maternal age. When 190 non-white epileptics were studied in the same way the same trend appeared but this time did not reach statistical significance. The authors considered the possibilities that this difference between whites and negroes is due (a) to the small size of the negro group or (b) to the negro children receiving more postnatal insults, but they did not then go on to examine the effect of other social factors on the relationship between prematurity and epilepsy. Douglas who was interested in the educational aspects of premature children found in his national survey of 5362 children, that premature children did less well than other children at school and were the subject of more adverse comments by teachers. However these differences were largely explained by the fact that premature birth is not only associated with poor living conditions but also low standards of maternal care. This same survey also found an association between prematurity and epilepsy (Cooper, 1965), and showed that more of the children without an obvious cause for their fits came from homes rated poorly for general standards of care, a finding which had previously been noted by Miller *et al.* (1960) in their survey of 1142 Newcastle children, where 7·7% were found to have suffered with convulsions during their first 5 years of life and where the strongest associations with these convulsions were acute infections and family inadequacy.

The implications of these studies are very important because one of the few well established general aetiological factors of delinquency and crime is the unfortunate upbringing of many of the individuals concerned. Consequently any association found between epilepsy and crime could be related to a common sociological variable such as the standard of maternal care.

Child battering which is an extreme example of poor maternal care illustrates very well the association between such low standards and brain damage. Kempe *et al.* (1962) in their classic paper on this problem reported their findings on 302 children who had clearly been attacked by their parents. Of these 33 had died and 85 had suffered permanent brain injury; in fact they noted that "subdural haematoma" (bleeding inside the skull) "with or without fracture of the skull is . . . an extremely frequent finding". Significantly the type of parent involved in this kind of case is frequently described as "psychopathic" with associated alcoholism, sexual promiscuity, marital instability and criminal convictions.

In the present survey, one boy seen in borstal, broke down in the middle of his interview and told of frequent beatings from his mother. He said he was convinced that his seizures were due to this as they only began in his teens after a particularly unpleasant episode when his mother had beaten him around the head with a leather strap until he was dazed. One or two other men talked of severe ear infections in childhood which had probably been neglected and even gone on to "meningitis" in one case.

Modelling, or learning by imitation seems to be a powerful force in determining our behaviour and attitudes. Perhaps, therefore, the handing on of constitutional weakness referred to earlier is, at least partly, the damaging of the next generation by both bad example and neglect. There is certainly a growing belief that this generation's battered will become next generation's batterers.

E. *Consequential Epilepsy*

Youngsters who, for whatever reason, grow up impulsive, reckless, careless and trouble prone, are of course particularly likely to end up in a criminal survey. This fifth hypothesis suggests that they are also a bit more likely than average to end up with cerebral damage. They may take foolish chances, drive recklessly, fail to care for themselves, and find themselves with an injury or illness.

"Len" came from a disturbed background, his parents continually rowing and separating until the final break when he was 9 years old. His mother described his childhood as punctuated by stealing, truancy, sleepwalking and recurrent nightmares, and at the age of 12 years he sustained his first conviction for stealing a lorry and was sent to an approved school. Following his release he was frequently in trouble but had had no suggestion of head injury or brain damage until the age of 17 years when just after joining the army he smashed up an army lorry and landed himself in hospital for two weeks with a mild head injury (full details unobtainable) but following this incident he began to complain of "fainting attacks" and was soon given his discharge on the grounds of "psychopathic personality". Although he had always refused to have an EEG there is little doubt that his "attacks" were epileptic in nature as they usually began with a pain behind the right eye which lasted for a minute or two until he fell to the ground convulsing his arms and legs. The frequency of these attacks was controlled in prison to 2 or 3 per year by the use of phenobarbitone. He resented the diagnosis 'epileptic' and was on the whole hostile to doctors whom he regarded as irritants rather than therapists. Clearly his criminality cannot mainly be attributed to the epilepsy or any underlying cerebral damage because the conviction came before the accident. It is much more reasonable to assume that his behaviour disorder led to reckless driving and the consequences mentioned. Even so the epilepsy had not helped him to stabilize and improve his behaviour.

"Michael" also illustrates this point. A dull man who could remember little of his early home life except that he didn't like it, he persistently wandered off, breaking away from his parents permanently at the age of eleven. His family (parents and grandparents) had always been "gypsies" moving about the countryside in caravans and so he received no schooling but was able to fend for himself by the age of eleven. As a boy he was frequently in trouble with the police for stealing, he soon learnt to drink heavily and received several drunkenness convictions. At the age of 24 he was involved in a pub brawl and received a serious blow to his head which caused a right frontal skull fracture. *Grand mal* epileptic seizures developed following this incident and he had had them ever since. Again his criminality (which has been increasing with the years) could hardly be attributed to his epilepsy, although it is significant to note that until the accident he could employ himself as a scrap dealer, whereas at the time of the interview he could not cope outside prison at all. The likeliest explanation is that a mixture of constitutional and environmental factors produced a personality with a behaviour disorder, this disorder led on to drinking and fighting and the epilepsy was consequent upon that; now that he has some cerebral damage he is less capable of managing then before and in any case will be regarded by others as unsuitable for employment, not only because he is erratic and steals but also because seizures afflict him about once a month which come without warning and which have resulted in moderately severe injuries on one or two occasions.

Interaction and Mixed Effects

Throughout this project both from the literature and the survey it has become increasingly evident that there are three main aspects of the relationship between epilepsy and antisocial behaviour
  (1) Early childhood environment and family pathology
  (2) Cerebral dysfunction
  (3) Attitudes, both of society, and of the individual (a) in response
        to his disorder and (b) in response to other people's attitudes
and that only occasionally can a prisoner's problems be assessed wholly or largely in terms of one of these areas. Usually there are marked interactions between all three.

This is hardly a new idea for although in the past workers have tended to concentrate upon *either* cerebral factors *or* the environment, there has been an increasing awareness and discussion of interaction in recent years. Bridge (1934, 1949) has suggested that their is a neurological substrate of epilepsy characterised by irritability and short attention span, and that as a result the epileptic interacts badly with his environment becoming intolerant, demanding and exhibiting temper tantrums. The environment, in its turn, begins to think of the child as endemically bad and the parents see the child as a trouble maker, "as time goes on, the child's way of reacting becomes set into a pattern, and elements of what is called 'the epileptic personality' appear".

In his important paper reviewing the psychiatric implications of brain damage in children Eisenberg (1957) pointed out that:

"Basic to an understanding of the clinical facts is the concept that the patient is a psychobiological entity, subject both to biological continuity of his own. The outcome of brain injury then, will be determined by factors operating in all these spheres. To begin with, one observes the quantitative and qualitative alterations in brain function produced by damage to its structure. On second level, the behaviour observed is influenced by the reorganisation of the previous personality of the patient in the face of his functional deficit. On still a third level, the social environment has a profound influence on the patient's performance — and, under certain conditions, the decisive influence. It is the interaction between these three classes of factors that determines the outcome in each particular case."

Birch *et al.* (1964) described, in some detail, the behavioural development of three brain damaged children and it is not difficult to infer with the authors, that the markedly different outcomes in the three cases was related to an interaction between the temperamental characteristics of the child, parental attitudes and practices, and the rest of the environment. They conclude that brain damage in childhood can lead to a whole host of consequences ranging from no apparent behavioural disturbance to serious disorganisation of social, intellectual and inter-personal functioning. Ounsted *et al.* (1966) are a little more specific and a little narrower in their interaction theory for the development of temporal lobe epilepsy. They suggest that birth injury may set up in some children a lesion which in later life potentiates seizures, the secondary seizures produce epileptic brain damage selectively in Ammon's horn (part of the temporal lobe) and hence lead to temporal lobe epilepsy. In his Icelandic survey of epilepsy Gudmundson could not attribute the mental changes of epileptics to any one cause; brain damage, inherited constitutions and socio-psychological influences all play their part.

Most of the case histories chosen so far have concentrated upon single cause and effect relationships. However they have all equally demonstrated the fundamental validity of the interaction hypothesis because never can any of the factors discussed be seen in total isolation. For most of the cases in the series it is impossible to sort out a particularly prominent aspect of relationship between the epilepsy and the behaviour which can usually only be viewed as a summation of factors. "Neil's" case illustrate this. He was adopted in early infancy by a childless middleclass couple. At first he did well at school and lived up to his father's high expectations but at the time of his change to secondary education his performance began to deteriorate, he became lethargic and complained of headaches. Eventually a brain tumour was discovered and removed. His recovery following the operation was slow and a post-operative one sided weakness never entirely disappeared; furthermore he developed epilepsy. He never completely regained his foothold at school and his father was disappointed. After leaving school at 15 he took a succession of menial jobs and he made several visits to hospital. The epilepsy, which he dreaded, did not improve and he attempted suicide and started to take amphetamines. Parental toleration of his problems and behaviour gradually fell until it finally collapsed altogether when he started to steal. The prison medical officer who reported on his case at his trial (for robbery) attributed his behaviour to brain damage, on the other hand his social worker regarded his behaviour as a reaction to rejection by those he counted on to support him in time of crisis. If one adds a third view that his behaviour was a reaction to the feelings of inadequacy, inferiority and horror which he expressed at interview and which stemmed from a comparison of his post-operative self image with his pre-morbid self image, the picture is almost complete. (A geneticist might point out that we know nothing of his blood relatives and he may have been the product of two disturbed personalities each of which had handed on a little of their own constitutional inferiority.) Which viewpoint is correct? Is it not likely that all three are correct, with each concept adding to the others and circular effects being inevitable?

Alcohol

No survey of any kind of criminal activity is complete without mentioning alcohol because it plays such a prominent part in a great deal of aberrant human behaviour. The astonishing lack of attention given to this fact by Parliament is perhaps an indication of how "serious" we all are about crime control. Chapter 5 has already indicated how important the alcohol factor might be in epileptic criminals. It could for example be possible for some alcoholics to be included in this survey because of recurrent withdrawal fits, but they did not in fact do so. Attention was drawn to one case ("Colin") in which alcohol clearly precipitated epileptic-like discharges in the EEG, but perhaps "Oscar" was a more typical example of the relationship between alcohol, epilepsy and anti-social behaviour found in this series, which can be regarded as another kind of interaction effect. Born thirteenth to poor parents, his father died before he was one year old. At the age of 9 years he was evacuated to another family and his mother died soon afterwards. The cause of his epilepsy and its date of onset is not known with accuracy but probably occurred in his teens. In spite of regular medication with phenobarbitone and phenytoin in prison he still had at least one *grand mal* seizure a month. He had always found life too difficult for him and had failed to keep any job for more than a few weeks at a time. He soon turned to drink for solace and by his mid thirties (at interview) was a skid-row, crude spirit drinking alcoholic. *En route* his general physical dilapidation had brought him tuberculosis and two stiff hips. He had had countless minor convictions for drunkenness offences and eight indictable offences for various kinds of stealing. The prisoner regarded his epilepsy as a considerable handicap to his rehabilitation and possible future employment and he may well have been correct as all attempts to admit him to after-care hostels had been unsuccessful because of his seizures. The prison doctor looking after him regarded his epilepsy as considerably exacerbated by his alcoholism, especially when outside prison; another arguable point of view.

No examples of overt brain damage caused by alcohol were noted in this sample, the only brain damaged alcoholic again illustrates the interaction effects available. "Peter" was an ex-police officer who had had a successful career for some years and a happy marriage. At the age of 36 he suffered a blow to his head in the left parietal region which caused a temporary (one month) paralysis to his right arm and leg. He left the police force and joined the army during the second world war, but when he complained of symptoms referrable to his right side the neurologist thought that "there is probably an hysterical perpetuation of the weakness". A year or two later he left the army and lost his wife much about the same time, following this he became depressed and began to drink heavily. He gradually deteriorated over the next 20 years to a meths-drinking, skid-row alcoholic. When he was sixty epileptic seizures appeared for the first time and as a result of one of these he was taken to hospital. At first the medical staff were inclined to view this new development as an example of "rum fits" (alcoholic withdrawal fits) but an air encephalogram x-ray showed marked cerebral atrophy mainly affecting the left hemisphere and mostly confined to the frontal region. Would he have developed the later atrophy if he had not suffered an earlier head injury? Did the effects of the injury or the loss of his wife drive him to drink? Did the alcoholism accelerate or cause the cerebral atrophy? Are the seizures alcoholic withdrawal fits or part of the atrophic syndrome? Decisive answers cannot be given to these questions partly because each of the concepts probably contains some of the truth.

Is Prison Appropriate?

Turning now from the possible relationships between epilepsy and crime to the issue of whether epileptics should be in prison at all the discussions become even more complex. Why is anybody sent to prison? Because they have committed an offence which merits that kind of punishment. So prison is punishment. However prisons are also institutions and have similarities to hostels, mental hospitals and the like, so perhaps prisons are more than just places of punishment. Indeed, the standard answer to this dilemma is that the punishment of imprisonment is being sent there and losing liberty; during imprisonment rehabilitation takes place. If general rehabilitation, then why not medical rehabilitation for epileptics? Why not indeed if it was appropriate to send the epileptics to prison in the first place. At no point is it possible to escape from the fact that prison sentences are punishments doled out by courts partly on a tariff basis. As the Streatfield Committee indicated, the 3 elements of a court sentence are (i) the tariff according to culpability, (ii) deterrence, (iii) correction or reform. When assessing culpability the court tries to assess "responsibility". If an epileptic were to commit an offence during a fit or unconscious phase with no premeditation of his behaviour whatsoever, then he will almost certainly be found not guilty, or if technically guilty, then not punishable. As can be seen from Chapter 4 such events are rare but the examples given in this discussion chapter lend strength to the argument that culpability can be reduced by the disease in an epileptic. It would simply be unjust to punish the brain damaged ex-policeman ("Peter") or even the epileptic young robber ("Neil") to the same extent as healthy men who commit identical offences. On the other hand a court may believe that prison offers the best opportunity to a man for reform. It's difficult to believe that the court sentenced "Peter" on this basis and in this instance punishment and deterrence (in the form of containment) must have been the only factors considered.

In spite of the fact that many of the staff spoken to felt that epileptics should never or only rarely be sent to prison, this survey indicates that for many of the epileptics prison acted as a clinic where they could have a limited amount of investigation, regular medication and a regular life (see p. 24). For this group, largely the homeless disorganised rootless men, the prisons provided a real medical service. In many ways of course this is a serious criticism of the National Health Service which ought to be able to offer facilities to precisely this group of men.

For the better integrated epileptic — a man, for example, who has worked out a daily routine to suit himself, who has been thoroughly investigated and who is prepared to take a few calculated risks on his own behalf. prison can be a terrible punishment. He falls to the bottom of the social hierarchy as an "eppy". At the time of the survey epileptics were forbidden to wear ties (because of their extra suicidal risk) whereas all other prisoners had to wear ties, so they were instantly recognisable. Most of the sample were "located flat" (i.e. not allowed to climb any stairs in the prison in case they had a fit) and were on restricted labour so that they avoided all contact with machinery and hot things. Some of these practices have changed recently but interestingly, at the time, the officer staff were on the whole very critical of the restrictions. A Principal Officer said "An epileptic is immediately restricted in all his activities and they are often just the people who need most help. It seems pointless and unfair. Why can't they be sent to open prisons where good training facilities are offered?" Another experienced PO said "Epileptics should not all be branded as unfit for No. 1 Labour, most of them could do it adequately. We're overcautious here, *all* epileptics are located flat and not allowed to work with machinery or ladders. The prize example was when we put these restrictions on an epileptic prisoner who was a steeple-jack by trade". An ordinary hospital officer observed "the special treatment (i.e. reduced work capacity) leads to boredom and this seems to cause more fits". A Chief Officer summed it up "By these restrictions we are protecting both the man and ourselves because we are liable for damages and compensation if he injures himself". Nevertheless not all voices were in unison. "There are distinct advantages to be an epileptic in prison — they can use 'epilepsy' as an excuse whenever they are in trouble. It's easy for them to scive off work." "They seem to be a particular sort of individual, always needing attention, always playing on the epilepsy." "You couldn't remove the label of epilepsy from them because it is they themselves who flaunt it about." "They do not mix well with other prisoners mainly because at the moment they earn less money. If their money was put up this wouldn't be fair work for work. It is better if they work in segregated conditions for 2 reasons (i) if they have a fit in public they frighten the other men and then there is always the danger of a riot breaking out (ii) when unconscious they will be stripped of all their belongings by the other prisoners. The best answer would be to segregate them to two specially designated prisons where they are not different from the other prisoners and where they can get specialist attention".

As stressed earlier prisons are only one kind of institution and therefore cannot be considered entirely in isolation from all other institutions. Certainly grave difficulties are posed for prison staff by an intermingling of penal, social, and medical functions. "Many of these men are not proper criminals at all". "We just act as nurse-maids". They understand well enough that when a man goes to prison for punishment they have a responsibility to care for him properly, and that includes providing essential medical treatment. What confuses them is the apparent failure of "society" to provide any alternative supportive service for the group whose main need is institutional care. All institutions surround themselves with admission criteria. In the early part of this century hysterical symptoms such as loss of function in limbs, or psychogenic fits were popular and effective ways of getting into mental hospitals. Nowadays the keys to the hospital door are overdoses and tension headaches. Prisons demand some form of law breaking activity before admission is allowed. Some epileptics who need institutional care use all these methods to gain entry to an appropriate place of shelter. Two pressures tend to force this group to explore the prison avenue more and more frequently. Firstly there is an overall diminution in the number of sheltered places of accommodation taking place, secondly once the prison road has been explored at all it is increasingly difficult to find alternative accommodation in non penal institutions which are usually able to select the clients they want and don't give special priority to ex-prisoners or criminals.

In 1961, Mr Enoch Powell, then Minister of Health, set out a 15 year plan to reduce the number of psychiatric beds in Britain by half and he hoped that most patients would receive treatment, not in mental hospitals but in psychiatric wings of general hospitals. He went on "Now look and see what are the implications of these bold words. They implying nothing less than the elimination of by far the greater part of this country's mental hospitals as they stand today . . . There they stand, isolated, majestic, imperious, brooded over by the gigantic water-tower and chimney combined, rising unmistakable and daunting out of the countryside — the asylums which our forefathers built with such immense solidity. Do not for a moment underestimate their power of resistance to our assault". Almost 15 years later they still temerariously survive, but a great change has been wrought. The concept of asylum, shelter, has gone from the Health Service. This is now to be provided (as indeed it was originally) by the local authorities using a system of hostels and the somewhat nebulous concept of "community care". Almost by definition the community doesn't care too much about the mad, the bad, and other stigmatised groups. One can imagine the enthusiastic reception with which the local ratepayers association and the local residents association would greet a proposal to establish a hostel for homeless ex-prisoner epileptics in their area (but see the footnote below).

The lack of community care and the run down of the mental hospitals are the biggest factors putting extra pressure on the prison system. This pressure is also reflected in the large and growing numbers of men currently using the incredibly inadequate facilities provided by local authorities for the homeless. In 1972 Tidmarsh and Wood surveyed the largest London reception centre which is provided by the Ministry of Social Security to give temporary accommodation to persons "without a settled way of life". At the time of the survey 4000 men new to the centre and 4000 old cases visited each year, with approximately 800 being accommodated on any one night. 42% of the new cases had convictions for indictable offences and 79% of the old cases had such convictions. About 1200 of the men visiting the centre were classified as mentally ill or mentally subnormal, 2500 were regarded as alcoholic, 2200 as personality disordered, 2200 men were classified as psychiatrically normal. The authors found that men with no psychiatric abnormalities were the least likely to have convictions.

In his thesis Tidmarsh (1975) elaborates on the special problems of the epileptics among this destitute population. Using the criteria set out in this book they found 10 epileptic men among 359 cases reviewed, a prevalence of 27·9/1000 which is 6 times the College of General Practitioners rate and 4 times the rate found in the prison survey here. As Tidmarsh points out this enormous difference with other surveys may be due to the inevitable underestimation of many of them but it is clearly way beyond the general population figure. As Tidmarsh indicates there is probably a real association between epilepsy and social failure, as measured in his case by destitution and in the present study by conflict with the law.

An interesting similarity between the epileptics in Camberwell reception centre and the prisoner epileptics is the high incidence of *grand mal* fits recorded. Nine out of the ten Camberwell epileptics had regular *grand mal* seizures. Eight of the ten had a criminal record and had served prison sentences, three had been in epileptic colonies, five in psychiatric or subnormality hospitals.

Many prison medical officers met in the course of this research stated that in their opinion the biggest single factor which confronted the epileptic prisoner was his release date because at that moment, unless he was one of the fortunate minority with family ties he would become homeless and be especially ill-equipped to survive in the accommodation rat race because of his dual handicap. Certainly after the research interview some of the subjects went on to talk of their own plight and often stressed the extreme difficulty of finding work and accommodation. In other words one of the biggest failures of our penal system so far as the epileptic is concerned (and possibly other handicapped groups also) is community care, or the lack of it. Community care, you may think, is not the responsibility of the penal system. Therein lies the dilemma.

FOOTNOTE

I was sufficiently impressed, during the course of this research, in the problem of post prison accommodation for the epileptic that I decided to develop an experimental project to see if this could be remedied. After the study was over therefore I sought advice from the National Association for the Care and Resettlement of Offenders (NACRO). At that time they didn't have much experience in the type of project I sought but they did two things. Firstly they sat round the table with me and helped thrash out a possible hostel scheme, secondly, they put me in touch with the Royal London Aid Society who run a series of hostels for ex-prisoners and other offenders. The Royal London Aid took the embryo scheme under its wing and the usual uphill struggle to get funds and suitable premises began. After several years we gathered sufficient money and found a house that a local authority would allow us to rent and where there was no local opposition to our scheme.

At the present time we have accommodation for 6 or 7 epileptic men, mostly in single rooms in what amounts to supervised digs. The project is run by a small house committee of interested professionals. They employ a non-residential social worker, a part-time cook, and a part-time cleaner. All 3 employees are women with family commitments outside the project. This means that they bring to the home an abundance of domestic skill and motherliness, things which our residents are very short of; it also means that for long periods, for example at night, weekends, and holiday times, the residents have to run their own lives entirely, make short term decisions and see what happens. This lack of supervision for some periods followed by close supervision at other times, together with a regular forum to discuss problems gives, in our opinion, a reasonable opportunity for institutionalised men to find some independence and learn some of the complex social skills society demands of them.

Most of our men are considerably handicapped socially (e.g. few of them work, few of them have family ties), clearly we cannot take individuals who need in-patient nursing for their epilepsy, or who are so disruptive that they cannot live in a group at all. Even so we are by no means short of suitable prospective clients. We do not have a policy concerning length of stay. A few leave because they find that the pressures of group living are irksome after a while. We hope we have, for them, been a useful oasis. Others find giving up their antisocial habits too big a price and get into trouble with the police. Still others want to remain and they regard the hostel as a permanent home. We encourage them to think like this as we believe the more usual policy of moving everyone round in an expensive game of musical hostels produces its own counterproductive tensions.

At the time of writing the project has only been operational for 18 months and no formal research has been built into it, although we intend to remedy that soon, but we are convinced that our early experience has demonstrated a need for this type of accommodation, and that there are ways of providing it agreeably on a low cost basis. We hope our neighbours agree that such a home does not spell disaster for a residential area, indeed one local has remarked that smartening up our property may have an improving effect on the neighbourhood. As always our biggest anxiety relates, in a time of severe inflation, to money, but to bore you further on that score would be presumptuous in a book of this sort.

J.C.G.

References

Alstrom, C. H. (1950) "Epilepsy", *Acta Psychiatric et Neurologica Scandinavica*, Supp. 63.

Bagley, C. R. (1971) *The Social Psychology of the Child with Epilepsy*, London: Routledge and Kegan Paul.

Bailey, N. J. (1959) *Statistical Methods in Biology*, London: EUP.

Banay, R. S. (1942) "Alcoholism and Crime", *Quarterly Journal of Studies in Alcoholism*, **2**, 686-716.

Barande, R. (1958) "L'etat dangereux chez les epileptiques", *Bulletin Societe Internationale de Criminologie*.

Bax, M. and MacKeith, R. (1963) *Minimal Cerebral Dysfunction*, London: Heinemann.

Beard, A. W. and Slater, E. (1962) "Schizophrenic-like Psychoses of Epilepsy", *Proceedings of the Royal Society of Medicine*, **55**, 311-14.

Birch, H., Thomas, A. and Chess, S. (1964) "Behavioural Development in Brain-Damaged Children", *Archives of General Psychiatry*, **11**, 596-603.

Bluglass, R. S. *A Psychiatric Study of Scottish Prisoners*, M.D. Thesis (unpublished).

Bowden, P. (1975) "Liberty and Psychiatry", *British Medical Journal*, **4**, 94-6.

Brewis, H., Poskarizer, D., Holland, C. and Miller, H. (1966) "Neurological Disease in an English City", *Acta Neurologica Scandinavica*, Supp. 24.

Bridge, E. M. (1934) "Mental State of the Epileptic Patient", *Archives of Neurology and Psychiatry*, **32**, 723-36.

Bridge, E. M. (1949) *Epilepsy and Convulsive Disorders in Children*, New York: McGraw Hill.

Brown, W. T. and Solomon, C. I. (1942) "Delinquency and the Electroencephalograph", *American Journal of Psychiatry*, **98**, 499-503.

Burt, C. (1944) *The Young Delinquent*, London: UCP.

Carter, J. D. (1947) "Children's Expressed Attitudes Toward their Epilepsy", *Nervous Child*, **6**, 34-7.

Cattell, R. B. (1948) *A Guide to Mental Testing*, London: ULP.

Caveness, W. F., Merritt, H. H., Gallup, G. H. and Ruby, E. H. (1965) "A Survey of Public Attitudes Towards Epilepsy in 1964", *Epilepsia*, **6**, 75-86.

Clark, L. P. (1914) "A Personality Study of the Epileptic Constitution", *American Journal of Medical Science*, **148**, 729-38.

Clark, L. P. (1918) "The True Epileptic, *New York Medical Journal*, **107**, 817-24.

Clark, L. P. (1925) "Some Psychological Data Regarding the Interpretation of Essential Epilepsy", *Journal of Nervous and Mental Diseases*, **61**, 51-9.

Cloward, R. A. and Ohlin, L. E. (1961) *Delinquency and Opportunity*, Glencoe: The Free Press.

College of General Practitioners (1960) "A Survey of the Epileptics in General Practice", *British Medical Journal*, ii, 416-22.

Cooper, J. E. (1965) "Epilepsy in a Longitudinal Survey of 5000 children", *British Medical Journal*, i, 1020-2.

Cowie, J., Cowie, V. and Slater, E. (1968) *Delinquency in Girls*, London: Heinemann.

Davison, K. and Bagley, C. R. (1969) "Schizophrenia-like Psychoses Associated with Organic Disorders of the Central Nervous System" in *Current Problems in Neuropsychiatry*, Ed. by R. N. Herrington, British Journal of Psychiatry Special Publication No. 4, Ashford, RMPA.

Delay, J., Deniker, P. and Barande, R. (1957) "Le Suicide des Epileptiques", *Encephale*, 46, 401-36.

Diethelm, O. (1934) "Epileptic Convulsions and the Personality Setting", *Archives of Neurology and Psychiatry*, 31, 755-67.

Douglas, J. W. B. (1960) "Premature Children at Primary Schools", *British Medical Journal*, i, 1008-13.

East, W. N. (1927) *An Introduction to Forensic Psychiatry in the Criminal Courts*, London: Churchill.

Edwards, G., Hensman, C. and Peto, J. (1971) "Drinking Problems amongst Recidivist Prisoners", *Psychological Medicine*, 1, 388-99.

Eisenberg, L. (1957) "Psychiatric Implications of Brain Damage in Children", *Psychiatric Quarterly*, 31, 72-92.

Ferguson, T. (1952) *The Young Delinquent in his Social Setting*, London: O.U.P.

Ferrero, G. L. (1911) *Criminal Man*, New York.

Fox, J. T. (1939) "Epileptics in the Community", *Journal of Mental Science*, 85, 940-52.

Frankenstein, C. (1959) *Psychopathy*, New York: Grune.

Gastaut, H. (1953) "So-Called Psychomotor and Temporal Epilepsy", *Epilepsia*, 2, 59-76.

Gastaut, H., Caveness, W. F., Landoct, H., Lorentz de Haas, A. M., McNaughton, F. L., Magnus, O., Merlis, J. K., Pond, D. A., Radermecker, J. and Storm van Leeuwen, W. (1964) "A Proposed International Classification of Epileptic Seizures", *Epilepsia*, 5, 297-306.

General Register Office (1960) *Classification of Occupations*, London: HMSO.

General Register Office (1964) *Census 1961—England and Wales*, London: HMSO.

Gibbens, T. C. N. and Prince, J. (1962) *Shoplifting*, London: ISTD:

Gibbens, T. C. N. and Silberman, M. (1970) "Alcoholism among Prisoners", *Psychological Medicine*, 1, 73-8.

Glaser, D. and Rice, K. (1959) "Crime, Age and Employment", in *The Sociology of Crime and Delinquency*, Ed. by M. Wolfgang, L. Savitz and N. Johnston, New York, Wiley.

Glass, D. V. (1954) *Social Mobility in Britain*, London: RKP.

Gordon, N. and Russell, S. (1958) "The Problem of Unemployment among Epileptics", *Journal of Mental Science*, 104, 103-14.

Goring, C. (1913) *The English Convict*, London: HMSO.

Gowers, W. R. (1881) *Epilepsy and Other Chronic Convulsive Diseases*, Reprinted by Dover Publications, New York 1964.

Graham, P. and Rutter, M. (1968) "Organic Brain Dysfunction and Child Psychiatric Disorder", *British Medical Journal*, iii, 695-700.

Greer, S., Gunn, J. C. and Koller, K. M. (1966) "Aetiological Factors in Attempted Suicide", *British Medical Journal*, **ii**, 1352-5.

Grunberg, F. and Pond, D. A. (1957) "Conduct Disorders in Epileptic Children" *Journal of Neurology, Neurosurgery and Psychiatry*, **20**, 65-8.

Gudmundsson, G. (1966) "Epilepsy in Iceland", *Acta Neurologica Scandinavica*, **43**, Supp. 25.

Guerrant, J., Anderson, W. W., Fischer, A., Weinstein, M. R., Jaros, R. M. and Deskins, A. (1962). *Personality in Epilepsy*, Springfield: Thomas.

Gunn, J. C. (1974) "Prison, Shelters, and Homeless Men", *Psychiatric Quarterly*, **48**, 505-12.

Gunn, J. and Fenton, G. (1971) "Epilepsy, Automatism, and Crime", *Lancet*, **i**, 1173-6.

Healy, W. (1929) *The Individual Delinquent*, Boston: Little, Brown, & Co.

Hecaen, H. and de Ajuriaguerra, J. (1956) *Troubles Mentaux au cours de Tumeurs Intracraniennes*, Paris: Masson.

Henriksen, B., Juul-Jensen, P. and Lund, M. (1970) "The Mortality of Epileptics", in *Life Assurance Medicine. Proceedings of the 10th International Congress of Life Assurance Medicine, London 1970* pp. 139-48, Ed. by R. D. C. Brackenridge, London: Pitman.

Hill, D. (1957) "Epilepsy", *British Encyclopaedia of Medical Practice*, 86-99.

Hill, D. (1959) "The Difficult Epileptic in his Social Environment", *Transactions of the Association of Industrial Medical Officers*, **9**, 46-50.

Hill, D. (1963) "Epilepsy: Clinical Aspects" in *Electroencephalography* ed. by D. Hill and G. Parr, London: MacDonald.

Hill, D. and Pond, D. A. (1952) "Reflections on One Hundred Capital Cases Submitted to Electroencephalography", *Journal of Mental Science*, **98**, 23-43.

Himler, L. E. and Raphael, T. (1945) "Follow-up Study on 93 College Students with Epilepsy", *American Journal of Psychiatry*, **101**, 760-3.

Home Office (1967) *Criminal Statistics (England and Wales) 1966*, London: HMSO.

Ingram, T. T. S. (1966) "Chronic Brain Syndromes in Childhood other than Cerebral Palsy, Epilepsy, and Mental Defect", in *Minimal Cerebral Dysfunction*, Ed. by M. Bax and R. MacKeith, London: Heinemann.

Isbell, H., Fraser, H. F., Wickler, A., Belleville, R. E. and Eisenman, A. J. (1955) "An Experimental Study of the Aetiology of Rum Fits and Delirium Tremens", *Quarterly Journal of Studies in Alcohol*, **16**, 1.

Jackson, H. (1890) "On Convulsive Seizures", *British Medical Journal*, **i**, 703, 765, and 821.

Jarvie, H. F. (1954) "Frontal Lobe Wounds Causing Disinhibition", *Journal of Neurology, Neurosurgery and Psychiatry*, **17**, 14-32.

Jarvie, H. F. (1958) "The Frontal Lobes and Human Behaviour", *Lancet*, **ii**, 365-8.

Jasper, H. and Kershman, J. (1941) "Electroencephalographic Classification of the Epilepsies", *Archives of Neurology and Psychiatry*, **45**, 903-43.

Jasper, H. and Kershman, J. (1949) "Classification of the EEG in Epilepsy", *Electroencephalography and Clinical Neurophysiology*, Supp. 2, 123-31.

Jones, J. G. (1965) "Employment of Epileptics", *Lancet*, **ii**, 486-9.

Juul-Jensen, P. (1964) "Epilepsy: A Clinical and Social Analysis of 1020 Adult Patients with Epileptic Seizures", *Acta Neurologica Scandinavica*, **40**. Supp. 5.

Kaila, M. (1942) "Uber die Durchschmittschaufigkeit der Geisterkrankheiten und des Schwachsinns in Finnland", *Acta Psychiatrica et Neurologica Scandinavica*, Supp. 17 47-67.

Kempe, C. H., Silverman, F. N., Steele, B. S., Droegemueller, W. and Silver, H. K. (1962) "The Battered Child Syndrome", *Journal of the American Medical Association*, 181, 17, 24.

Kiørbe, E. (1954) "Kriminalitet blandt Epileptikere", *Nord T.f. Kriminal videnskab*, 42, 35-48.

Kligman, D. and Goldberg, D. A. (1975) "Temporal Lobe Epilepsy and Aggression", *Journal of Nervous and Mental Disease*, 160, 324-41.

Knobloch, H. and Pasamanick, B. (1966) "Prospective Studies on the Epidemiology of Reproductive Casualty: Methods, Findings and Some Implications", *Merrill-Palmer Quarterly*, 12, 27-43.

Knox, S. J. (1968) "Epileptic Automatism and Violence", *Medicine, Science, and the Law*, 8, 96-104.

Krohn, W. (1961) "Epilepsy in Northern Norway", *Acta Psychiatrica et Neurologica Scandinavica*, 36, Supp. 150, 215-25.

Krohn, W. (1963) "Causes of Death Among Epileptics", *Epilepsia*, 4, 315-21.

Kurland, L. T. (1959/60) "The Incidence and Prevalence of Convulsive Disorders in a Small Urban Community", *Epilepsia*, 1, 143-61.

Lancet (1953) "The Epileptic Child" (Annotation), ii, 387.

Lees, F. (1967) "Alcohol and the Nervous System", *Hospital Medicine*, 2, 264-70.

Lennox, W. G. (1942) "Mental Defect in Epilepsy and the Influence of Heredity", *American Journal of Psychiatry*, 98, 733-9.

Lennox, W. G. and Lennox, M. A. (1960) *Epilepsy and Related Disorders*, (2 Vols) Boston: Little, Brown & Co.

Lennox, W. G. and Markham, C. H. (1953) "The Sociopsychological Treatment of Epilepsy", *Journal of the American Medical Association*, 152, 1690-4

Lesser, A. J. and Hunt, E. P. (1954) "The Nation's Handicapped Children", *American Journal of Public Health*, 44, 166-70.

Lilienfield, A. M. and Pasamanick, B. (1954) "Association of Maternal and Fetal Factors with the Development of Epilepsy", *Journal of the American Medical Association*, 155, 719-24.

Lishman, W. A. (1968) "Brain Damage in Relation to Psychiatric Disability after Head Injury", *British Journal of Psychiatry*, 114, 373-410.

Lishman, W. A. (1973) "The Psychiatric Sequelae of Head Injury: A Review", *Psychological Medicine*, 3, 304-18.

Logan, W. P. D. and Cushion, A. A. (1958) *Studies on Medical and Population Subjects No. 14. Morbidity Statistics from General Practice*, Vol. I (General) GRO. London: HMSO.

Lombroso, C. (1889) *L'Uomo Delinquente*, Turin: Bocca.

Lorentz de Haas, A. M. (1960) "Epilepsy and Criminality", *Address to the 4th International Criminological Congress*, The Hague.

MacDonald, J. M. (1969) *Psychiatry and the Criminal*, Springfield: Thomas.

McCord, W. and McCord, J. (1956) *Psychopathology and Delinquency*, New York: Grune and Stratton.

Matheson, J. C. M. and Hill, D. (1943) "Electroencephalography in Medico-legal Problems" *Medico-legal and Criminological Review*, 11, 173-81.

Maudsley, H. (1873) *Body and Mind,* London: MacMillan.

Maudsley, H. (1906) *Responsibility in Mental Disease — 6th Edn,* London: Kegan Paul, Trench, Trubener and Co.

Maxwell, A. E. (1961) *Analysing Qualitative Data,* London: Methuen.

Mignone, R. J., Donnelly, E. F. and Sadowsky, D. (1970) "Psychological and Neurological Comparisons of Psychomotor and Non-psychomotor Epileptic Patients", *Epilepsia,* 11, 345-59.

Miller, F. J. W., Court, S. D. H., Walton, W. S. and Knox, E. G. (1960) *Growing-up in Newcastle-upon-Tyne,* London: OUP.

Miller, H. (1961) "Accident Neurosis", *British Medical Journal,* i, 919-25 and 992-8.

Miller, H. (1966) "Mental Sequelae of Head Injury", *Proceedings of the Royal Society of Medicine,* 59, 257-61.

Ministry of Health (1956) *Sub-Committee on the Medical Care of Epileptics,* London: HMSO.

Morris, T. and Blom-Cooper, L. (1964) *A Calendar of Murder,* London: Joseph.

Notkin, J. (1928) "Is there an Epileptic Personality Make-Up?", *Archives of Neurology and Psychiatry,* 20, 799-803.

O'Connell, B. A. (1960) "America and Homicide", *British Journal of Delinquency,* 10, 262-76.

Ounsted, C., Lindsay, J. and Norman, R. (1966) *Biological Factors in Temporal Lobe Epilepsy,* London: Spastics Society — Heinemann.

Penfield, W. and Jasper, H. (1954) *Epilepsy and the Functional Anatomy of the Human Brain,* London: Churchill.

Penfield, W. and Kristiansen, K. (1951) *Epileptic Seizure Patterns,* Springfield: Thomas.

Penrose, L. S. (1939) "Mental Disease and Crime: Outline of a Comparative Study of European Statistics", *British Journal of Medical Psychology,* 18, 1-13.

Pinel, P. (1806) (Translated by D. D. Davies — 1962) *A Treatise on Insanity,* New York: Hafner.

Pond, D. A. (1957) "Psychiatric Aspects of Epilepsy", *Journal of the Indian Medical Profession,* 3, 1441-51.

Pond, D. A. (1961) "Psychiatric Aspects of Epileptic and Brain-Damaged Children", *British Medical Journal,* ii, 1377-82, and 1454-9.

Pond, D. A. and Bidwell, B. H. (1960) "A Survey of Epilepsy in Fourteen General Practices. II. Social and Psychological Aspects", *Epilepsia,* 1, 285-99.

Pond, D. A., Bidwell, B. H. and Stein, L. (1960) "A Survey of Epilepsy in Fourteen General Practices. I. Demographic and Medical Data", *Psychiatrica, Neurologica, Neurochirurgia,* 63, 217-36.

Prudhomme, C. (1941) "Epilepsy and Suicide", *Journal of Nervous and Mental Diseases,* 94, 722-31.

Pruyser, P. W. (1953) "Psychological Testing in Epilepsy", *Epilepsia* (3rd series), 2, 23-36.

Roth, M. (1968) "Cerebral Disease and Mental Disorders of Old Age as Causes of Antisocial Behaviour" in *The Mentally Abnormal Offender,* London: Ciba Foundation.

Rutter, M., Tizard, J. and Whitmore, K. (1970) *Education, Health, and Behaviour,* London: Longman.

Rylander, G. (1939) *Personality Changes after Operations on Frontal Lobes*, Copenhagen: Munksgaard.

Schneider, K. (1958) (Translated by M. W. Hamilton 1959) *Clinical Psychopathology*, 5th Edition, New York.

Slater, E. and Roth, M. (1969) *Clinical Psychiatry (3rd Edn)*, London: Baillière, Tindall and Cassell.

Small, J., Hayden, M. and Small, I. (1966) "Further Psychiatric Investigations of Patients with Temporal and Non-temporal Lobe Epilepsy", *American Journal of Psychiatry*, **123**, 303-10.

Small, J., Milstein, V. and Stevens, J. (1962) "Are Psychomotor Epileptics Different?" *Archives of Neurology*, **7**, 187-94.

Stafford-Clark, D. and Taylor, F. H. (1949) "Clinical and Electroencephalographic Studies of Prisoners charged with Murder", *Journal of Neurology, Neurosurgery and Psychiatry*, **12**, 325-30.

Stein, C. (1933) "Hereditary Factors in Epilepsy", *American Journal of Psychiatry*, **89**, 989-1037.

Stevens, J. (1966) "Psychiatric Implications of Psychomotor Epilepsy", *Archives of General Psychiatry*, **14**, 461-71.

Streatfield Committee (1961) *Report of the Interdepartmental Committee on the Business of the Criminal Courts*, London: HMSO.

Sullivan, W. C. (1924) *Crime and Insanity*, London: Arnold.

Symonds, C. (1955) "Classification of the Epilepsies", *British Medical Journal*, **i**, 1235-8.

Taylor, D. C. and Falconer, M. A. (1968) "Changes in Clinical, Socio-economic and Psychological Adjustment after Temporal Lobectomy for Epilepsy", *British Journal of Psychiatry*, **114**, 1247-61.

Taylor, J. (1958) *Selected Writings of John Hughlings Jackson — Vol. 1*, New York: Hodder & Stoughton.

Temkin, O. (1945) *The Falling Sickness*, Baltimore: Johns Hopkins Press.

Thomas, D. S. (1925) *Social Aspects of the Business Cycle*, London: Routledge.

Tidmarsh, D. (1975) Psychiatric Disorder in a Population of Homeless Destitute Men — MD thesis — Cambridge.

Tidmarsh, D. and Wood, S. Personal Communication.

Tizard, B. (1962) "The Personality of Epileptics — a Discussion of the Evidence", *Psychological Bulletin*, **59**, 196-210.

Tuke, D. H. (1892) *A Dictionary of Psychological Medicine*, London: Churchill.

Ursin, H. (1960) "The Temporal Lobe Substate of Fear and Anger", *Acta Psychiatrica et Neurologica Scandinavica*, **35**, 378.

Victor, M. and Adams, R. D. (1953) "The Effect of Alcohol on the Nervous System", *Research Publications of the Association of Nervous and Mental Diseases*, **32**, 526-73.

Victor, M. and Brausch, C. (1967) "The Role of Abstinence in the Genesis of Alcoholic Epilepsy", *Epilepsia*, **8**, 1-20.

West, D. J. (1963) *The Habitual Prisoner*, London: Heinemann.

West, D. J. and Farrington, D. P. (1973) *Who Becomes Delinquent?* London: Heinemann.

Williams, D. (1953) "The Phenomena of Epilepsy", *British Medical Journal*, **i**, 173-6.

Wilson, W. P., Stewart, L. F. and Parker, J. B. (1959/60) "A Study of Socio-Economic Effects of Epilepsy", *Epilepsia*, **1**, 300-15.

Wolfgang, M. E. (1960) "Cesare Lombroso", in *Pioneers in Criminology*, Ed. by H. Mannheim, London: Stevens.

World Health Organisation (1957) *Juvenile Epilepsy—Report of a Study Group* (Technical Report No. 130), Geneva: WHO.

Yarrow, M. R., Campbell, J. D. and Burton, R. V. (1964) "Reliability of Maternal Retrospection", *Family Process*, **3**, 207-18.

Index